ACCLAIM

MW00845012

Status Quo Thinking Is Harming Your Health

"In the early months after founding Virta Health, we were struggling to find a clinical study site to determine the long-term safety of our virtual diabetes reversal program. Mainstream academia wanted nothing to do with us. At a symposium in Denver, a stranger stopped me and declared: 'Your research has changed the lives of many of my patients but some of them are seeing big increases in LDL cholesterol. Do you think this is safe?' Looking at her nametag, I parried: 'Dr. Hallberg, do you want to do a study to find out?' Her response: 'Hell yes!' The study was initially intended to last two years. In the following six years, Sarah's inspiration and dedication amazingly delivered a 465-person, 5-year long study that has seismically shifted diabetes care away from management to reversal. Her resulting peer-reviewed publications have been cited by our academic colleagues – yes, those prior skeptics - over a thousand times! Type 2 diabetes is now proven to be reversible, giving hope and renewed health to hundreds of millions. And Sarah – aptly a Florence Nightingale of the 21st century - played the critical role in this healthcare transformation."

– Steve Phinney, MD, PhD,
Professor of Medicine
emeritus, UC Davis,
Founder, Virta Health

"Sarah Hallberg leaves nothing on the table. This book is part heart-wrenching memoir, part indictment of our medical system, and a big part visionary road map for an enlightened healthcare system focused on the root causes of our chronic disease and diabetes epidemic. A must-read for anyone frustrated with our current medical paradigm and searching for a way of healing for us all."

– Mark Hyman, MD,
author of the #1 *New York Times* bestseller,
Young Forever

"We can't begin to do justice to all that Sarah meant to us as individuals, as patients, and as colleagues. She will be forever missed, but her mission for patient advocacy will live on in all of us. She has touched and inspired so many lives and we owe it to her, and to ourselves, to continue her mission."

– Bret Scher, MD, FACC,
President, Boundless Health

"Sarah Hallberg was one of the generals in the army that fights to overcome diabetes. Only God knows how many people she helped, but it must run into the millions. In enabling so many people to become healthy and live to old age, ironically Sarah's life was cut short by cancer. But in her relatively brief years she accomplished more good and helped more people than most could if they lived to be 109. There is something far more important than living to an old age, and that is to be a blessing to as many people as you can reach. Sarah surely reached many, and I pray that this latest book will be yet one more fruitful branch springing from her incredibly productive life."

– Dennis Pollock, Founder,
Beat Diabetes, YouTube
Channel

"I was impressed by her courage, scientifically speaking, in challenging the status quo in traditional diabetes guidelines."

– Saleh Aldasouqi, MD,
Professor of Medicine and
Chief of the Division of
Endocrinology,
Michigan State University

"Only troublemakers really make change. And Sarah was among the best of them!"

— Britt Volk, PhD, RD

"Dr. Hallberg was truly a pioneer in the fields of type 2 diabetes, obesity, and metabolic health. Her legacy as a physician and researcher lives on as her work reaches countless people who are reclaiming their health - *and their lives* - through her simple, down-to-earth, evidence-backed dietary advice."

— Amy Berger, MS, CNS, Author of *The Alzheimer's Antidote* and *End Your Carb Confusion*

"Dr. Hallberg was a pioneer and futurist who knew the critical value of scientific data. She saw what was essential to helping people and pushed to make that happen, often defying the odds. She was also deeply realistic. Read this book to appreciate the grit it takes to go against the tides and succeed in impacting public health and diabetes."

— Shamiram Feinglass, MD, MPH

"Sarah sparkled and her passion ignited hope and inspiration in others. Her quest for justice and healing moved mountains in treating diabetes and changed lives."

> — Warren Ng, MD,
> Aspen Global Leadership
> Network HIF3, The Justice
> League

"Dr. Sarah Hallberg was a bright light in this world who empowered thousands of patients to regain control of their health and reverse Type 2 diabetes through food. The field of metabolic health, and medicine as a whole, would not be where it is today without Dr. Hallberg's trailblazing efforts. She changed the world and diabetes care as we know it, and will continue to serve as a huge inspiration in our work and everything we do."

> — Victoria Field &
> Angela Poff, PhD,
> Co-Founders,
> Metabolic Health Initiative

"If medical training has left you questioning the status quo and wanting better for your patients and your own profession, this book will inspire you. If you have a fraction of Dr. Sarah Hallberg's optimism and sense of urgency, you will change healthcare for the better. The sadness I felt upon learning of Sarah's passing is lessened a bit knowing her life will have helped so many others. To borrow from a proverb: 'The star that burns twice as bright, burns half as long.' Dr. Sarah Hallberg will be remembered as one of the brightest stars in healthcare."

> – Eric C. Westman, MD MHS,
> Associate Professor of
> Medicine, Duke University
> Health System;
> Past President, Obesity
> Medicine Association

"In her final, groundbreaking work, Dr. Sarah Hallberg challenges the entrenched beliefs of modern medicine, urging readers to question the status quo for the sake of their health. This book is both a passionate plea and a testament to a life dedicated to healing. Published posthumously, this book serves as Hallberg's enduring legacy, calling for a radical shift in our approach to healthcare."

> – Peter Attia, MD, Founder,
> Early Medical

"Dr. Hallberg's unwavering determination set her apart; she refused to be a bystander in the realm of chronic disease and emerged as a resolute leader seeking innovative solutions. Her commitment to challenging the status quo and tirelessly pursuing effective, sustainable, and preventative approaches for managing diabetes was simply unparalleled.

"Dr. Hallberg exemplified authentic leadership, recognizing that we couldn't tackle these challenges in isolation. She passionately urged others to unite and collaborate, underlining the importance of our shared mission to create substantial change. Her enduring spirit and steadfast dedication continue to be a wellspring of inspiration for us all."

— Michael Giardina,
CrossFit Health

"Dr. Sarah Hallberg was a visionary leader in international metabolic health who had a unique ability to both deliver empathetic care to her many patients and, in mid-career, to take on leadership of a stunning clinical research program that has changed the way type 2 diabetes is understood and treated. In this book, *The Status Quo is Harming Your Health*, Sarah's energetic voice comes through as though she were still with us - from her ability to explain the complexities of medicine with simplicity to her fierce patient advocacy. Sarah not only clarifies a new path for so many to reverse their diabetes, but also tells the story of her own cancer treatment as she seeks to extend her life and cherish her time with family in the face of overwhelming odds."

– Dr. James McCarter,
Medical Director, Abbott
Laboratories; Adjunct
Professor,
Washington University
School of Medicine

"It has been an honor and inspiration to know Sarah. In her uniquely motivational style, Sarah chronicles her impressive professional journey as a physician fighting against the status quo as well as her personal battle with cancer. Sarah was simply a powerhouse of a person who motivated and elevated everyone around her. Anyone who reads her story will be moved to be a better person while learning valuable information about the science of managing diabetes with nutrition."

– Jeff S. Volek, PhD, RD,
Professor of Human
Sciences,
The Ohio State University,
Founder and Founding Chief
Science Officer, Virta Health

"Dr. Sarah Hallberg, relentless crusader in the fight against diabetes, constantly challenged conventional wisdom that prioritizes pharmaceutical solutions over dietary and lifestyle changes. With unwavering determination, she emphasized the transformative power of nutritional interventions, gifting us with an alternative path to wellness that, for the most part, is still overshadowed by mainstream approaches. Dr. Hallberg will remain a beacon of hope for countless individuals, underscoring the urgent need for a paradigm shift in diabetes treatment at a time when the world grapples with its escalating health consequences. Her pioneering work is a testament to the pivotal importance of the choices we make every day."

> – David Perlmutter, MD, FACN

"Her tireless efforts to help and teach others will continue for generations to come."

> – Vinnie Tortorich, Author, Podcaster, Documentarian

"Dr. Sarah Hallberg was a pioneer in educating the clinical community about the very important role of nutrition and lifestyle in reversing type 2 diabetes and controlling cardiometabolic risk factors. We at Cardiometabolic Health Congress (CMHC) were fortunate to have Dr. Hallberg speak at several of our meetings, where her unique insights on type 2 diabetes management were always a highlight. Dr. Hallberg will be missed by her CMHC colleagues, the entire cardiometabolic health community, and beyond."

– The CMHC Team

"Sarah was such a dynamic inspiring person. She pioneered the Virta Health study with amazing results, which has given great hope to people with type 2 diabetes. Low Carb Down Under has been privileged to publish six of her wonderful YouTube lectures. Sarah lives on in our memories."

– Rod Tayler,
Founder of LDCU

"For those of us fortunate enough to have known Sarah Hallberg, her independent thinking, willingness to take on heavily funded and entrenched authorities, sheer persistence, grace, and humanity have left an indelible mark. Her career evolution and work to reverse type 2 diabetes is hugely impactful for millions of patients, and her personal story doing all this while being a loving and supportive wife, mother and friend, all while bravely battling advanced stage lung cancer is truly inspirational. This book will change how you eat, how you think about established medical dogma, and how you live your life. Thank you, Sarah, for leaving this as part of your legacy."

> — Rushika Fernandopulle,
> M.D., M.P.P, Co-founder
> and former CEO, Iora Health

"Maya Angelou once said, 'I've learned that people will forget what you said, people will forget what you did, but people will never forget how you made them feel.' Sarah is different. I remember that Sarah was a fierce advocate for people with diabetes. She said, there is evidence you can be healthier and you deserve that, and then she made it happen. And once you got to know Sarah, you realized her advocacy didn't stop there — she was an advocate for anyone who deserved better. That advocacy of Sarah's was infectious and lives on today among people inspired by what she said and did, because above all, she made you feel as though you were a badass who could truly make a difference."

> — Amy McKenzie, colleague at Virta Health, and above all, friend

"Sarah Hallberg's life was a triumph of spirit and of science. Her remarkable book is the story of her groundbreaking research and her courageous mission to demonstrate that diabetes can be reversed with the right dietary choices. A must-read."

> – Gary Taubes, journalist and author of *Rethinking Diabetes*

"Sarah was a woman on a mission. She was a true force of nature with endless energy. No obstacle, no ask, no complex situation or no setback could slow her down. And I could tell the fuel driving her forward was pure selfless desire to help others, help people rid their chronic disease."

> – Sami Inkinen, CEO & Founder of Virta Health

"Dr. Sarah is my friend, Antigone sister, medicine woman, truth-teller and inspiration. In the five fighting years I had the privilege of knowing her, I will always remember the superhero energy she had for her work, patients and family. There was no stopping this woman! And with this book, she will continue to make an impact. Her legacy is eternal."

> – Saira

"Sarah Hallberg was a force of nature, a trailblazing physician, and a dedicated advocate for nutritional ketosis. Her initial work through the IUH clinical trial left an indelible mark in this field. Her research on nutritional ketosis and her role as the principal investigator of the IUH trial were the main pillars that helped found Virta Health through a science and evidence-based approach. Through her tireless efforts and motivation, she not only advanced scientific knowledge but also cared for many patients in her clinic using this nutritional approach. She inspired not only fellow physicians but also researchers who aspire to continue her work and passion. She was indeed a wonderful friend who has always been there for me. It is hard to imagine not having her around, but she will always be in our hearts forever."

— Shaminie J Athinarayanan, PhD, Associate Director of Clinical Research, Virta Health

"The world needs more Dr. Sarahs. She was an extraordinary doctor, the one who really brought type 2 diabetes reversal to public consciousness. Her 2015 TEDx talk was revolutionary. I saw it within a week of my own diagnosis of T2D. That same week I began my low-carbohydrate journey and I can say that she is right: Diabetes is reversible through diet.

"I saw first-hand her determination to continue the fight for those with T2D even when her own cancer diagnosis was sapping so much of her strength. There was no advocate more passionate for those who did not have their own megaphone. She inspired me to help empower people to understand – the condition, their options – for themselves.

"When Dr. Sarah knew she was dying, she embarked on writing this book, to ensure that even when she herself was no longer with us, she could still encourage both the medical profession and the public to think for themselves. She looked at the evidence and acted on it. Dr. Sarah did not accept the status quo. She thought differently. She thought for herself, not of herself. *The Status Quo Is Harming Your Health* is a powerful must-read."

> – Amanda Atkins, Founder, Afinia Films, Executive Producer, *Fat Fiction, The Diabetes Solution,* and *CanceRevolution*

Status Quo Thinking Is Harming Your Health

a physician's final plea

by

Dr. Sarah Hallberg

This publication contains the opinions and ideas of its author. It is sold with the understanding that the author and publisher are not engaged in rendering health services in the book. The reader should consult her or his own medical and health providers as appropriate before adopting any of the suggestions in this book or drawing references from it.

The author and publisher specifically disclaim all responsibility for any liability, loss or risk, personal or otherwise, which is incurred as a consequence, directly or indirectly, of the use and application of any of the contents of this book.

Copyright © 2024 by Olio LLC
Foreword copyright © 2024 by Nina Teicholz
Cover design by Jennifer Rider

to my family:

Brad,
who supported my career
and tended to me in sickness and in health

Noah, Ava, and Luna,
who embody your dad and me and also possess
so many amazing attributes of your own

…I will miss you all more than words can describe.

If you always do what you've always done, you always get what you've always gotten.

- Jessie Potter

Table of Contents

PART 3: CHANGE YOURSELF

Foreword

Pint-sized, with a shock of blond hair and blue eyes, Dr. Sarah Hallberg could easily impress you as the world's most vibrant soccer mom, the one who cheered the loudest from the sidelines and who consistently won the school cake-baking competitions. She was Mother Christmas, purchasing gifts months in advance and spending weeks creating elaborate wrappings. She had a passion that mixed whimsy with joy. And that same passion extended to helping people, not just her own family or her patients, but over the course of her astonishing career to the many millions of people suffering with type 2 diabetes. For them, she came to feel a special commitment. And for them, she helped pioneer a profound, transformative idea: that type 2 diabetes is not an intractable, progressive, hopeless condition. In fact, type 2 diabetes can be reversed.

"Dr. Sarah," as she was known, did not start off her career in medicine. A fitness devotee, she trained as an exercise physiologist; over time she realized that doctors had far greater influence on the prevention of disease, so she applied to medical school. She had a zeal for preventive medicine, and was impatient to overcome challenges. In this memoir, she describes how, during her medical training, she lasered her focus on an especially demanding supervisor, confronted him fearlessly and eventually earned his respect. This flair for winning over naysayers was a particular Sarah superpower. Her personal charisma together with a skill for explanation helped fuel her ideas, even controversial ones. No doubt this talent is one reason why as of this writing, over eleven million people have watched her TEDx talk on diabetes. Sarah was blessed with the drive to challenge the status quo and a unique ability to touch hearts and open minds.

However, even upon becoming a primary care doctor in her adopted home of West Lafayette, Indiana, Sarah's path forward remained unclear. After practicing internal medicine for nearly a decade, she realized that she was miserable. She said, "I would come home from work, put my head down and say, 'I'm *part* of the problem. I'm a legal drug dealer.'" Because, as she explained, all she did was write prescriptions and, far too often, "watch people get worse."

Luckily, when the University of Indiana Health Arnett asked her to open an obesity clinic, she was able to spend nearly a year investigating the complex scientific literature on obesity and diabetes. At the start of the project, she was a low-fat devotee, planning to counsel her patients to follow her lead in avoiding fat and counting calories. While researching the science, however, she was shocked: "I discovered there simply wasn't evidence to support what we're telling people!" By the time Sarah opened the clinic doors, she had landed on a low-carbohydrate approach to treating obesity. Shortly thereafter, she was surprised to find that beyond the significant weight loss her patients were experiencing, she saw their type 2 diabetes "go away." Her team was pulling patients off hundreds of units of insulin, often within a matter of weeks.

These revelations during the early days of her clinic set Dr. Sarah on a path that helped speed a change in diabetes treatment. In 2015, she teamed up with leading scientists in the field, including Stephen

Phinney and Jeff Volek, who had co-authored the seminal 2011 book, *The Art and Science of Low Carbohydrate Living,* which had been a major influence for her. Now, Steve and Jeff, along with Sami Inkinen, a co-founder of Trulia and former Ironman athlete, had recently started a company called Virta Health. Sami had been mystified to find that despite his arduous training, his blood sugar level indicated prediabetes, and he came to understand that even exercise could not undo the ill effects of excessive sugars and starches on the body. Sami, Steve, and Jeff wanted Virta to test the effectiveness of a very low-carbohydrate (ketogenic) diet, as well as a novel telemedicine approach to the delivery of type 2 diabetes health care. The goal would be not just management of diabetes, but reversal.

For these Virta founders, encountering Sarah was magic. They had been seeking to conduct a clinical trial that could establish high-quality evidence for their treatment, but were having trouble finding a lead investigator. They needed someone at a welcoming institution, plus access to a patient population. Sarah was that person. Not only did she have the necessary connections and community support, she had the tenacity to jump the many hurdles that Virta was sure to encounter along the way. Even so, the tiny team from Virta that landed in West Lafayette to help launch the trial, living out of suitcases in nearby hotels, could barely believe Sarah's sense of urgency. She was signing up subjects while the ink was still drying on the institutional approval forms.

The study that emerged is arguably the most important trial in the history of type 2 diabetes. For participants receiving the ketogenic treatment, it demonstrated dramatic decreases in blood sugar levels and diabetic medications, and significant weight loss. People were reversing out of diabetes. This was especially striking given how long the trial participants had been living with diabetes: on average, for eight-plus years, and some for more than 20. For a population coming from such an entrenched starting point, reversal is even more remarkable. Most other trials begin with populations that are far less sick, perhaps to boost the odds for success. Not this trial.

The Virta results were impressive, but because they dramatically upended status quo thinking, Sarah's team met with pushback from many diabetes and nutrition experts and organizations. To this day, some experts simply will not entertain these legitimate, evidence-based trial results because they contradict the status quo and threaten their reputations and livelihoods. Some experts are also subtly influenced by pharmaceutical interests which surely do not include an intervention that helps people eliminate medications.

In June 2022, the Virta team presented the trial's five-year results at a meeting of the American Diabetes Association. Only one other diet – the Mediterranean – has had positive results after five years, and those were exclusively on cardiovascular outcomes. The ketogenic diet is now the only other diet with such long-term outcomes. At Year 5, researchers – who no longer included Sarah – found that the ketogenic dieters maintained significant weight loss, lower blood sugars, and sustained reversal of their type 2 diabetes, while also keeping down their need for medications. Those in the standard-care/control group, however, continued to need ever-increasing amounts of medications.

Sarah would no doubt have been proud to see this outcome. She also would have been happy to see that the term "reversal," while still controversial, is being used more and more in the field. Although diabetes experts have tended to prefer the term "remission," since the condition will come back if a person reverts to eating high quantities of carbohydrates, she insisted on reversal, because people were successfully lowering their blood sugars to levels that reversed a diagnosis of type 2 diabetes.

Sarah was not around by the time of the ADA presentation because she died on March 28, 2022, at age 50, almost five years from the date in June 2017 that she collapsed, was rushed to the hospital, and diagnosed with stage 4 lung cancer that had metastasized to the brain. No, she never smoked. Nor was she around second-hand smoke. Despite the fatigue, nausea, pain, and other side effects of treatment, Sarah maintained her hectic work schedule, on a mission to convince the health establishment that type 2 diabetes does not have to be a chronic, progressively worsening, financially back-breaking disease. Sarah believed in hope. She wanted her patients to know that contrary to everything they'd been told for years or even decades, this disease from which they suffered was not a death sentence. She extended a ferocious force-field of protection around her patients, many of whom had been buffeted by the medical system and felt demoralized, and often despaired. She wanted to provide the compassion and care they needed, which partly involved giving people a sense of their autonomy and individual dignity. As much as anything, she wanted to give patients the right to choose. She gave her patients the facts – never talking down to them – and encouraged them to make their own dietary choices, modified by the low-carbohydrate approach.

In 2017, seeking to address the status quo at ever-higher levels, Sarah joined the fight to change the US Dietary Guidelines for Americans, the nation's top nutrition policy. In 2018, she gave a formal briefing to Congress on the topic of Food as Medicine, with a focus on diabetes and weight loss. In 2020 she flew to Washington, DC, to testify before the Dietary Guidelines Advisory Committee about the need for a low-carbohydrate approach in the Guidelines, and later – though her sickness was increasingly taking a toll on her – advocated for this policy to be more tailored to the individual needs of different cultural, ethnic, and socioeconomic groups. This was all part of her passionate effort in her final years to push for greater equity in healthcare – for all people. She also became active in the Nutrition Coalition, a group which I founded and is devoted to ensuring that our country's nutrition policy is evidence-based; she signed on as both a board member and Chair of the Scientific Council.

Sarah will be remembered for how she could light up a room and the way her relentless, revved-up dynamism beamed a thousand watts. She was a compassionate, selfless, and dedicated human being: a fighter for love, healing, equity – and evidence-based science. She will remain an inspiration. May her legacy, a world in which reversing type 2 diabetes is possible, live on.

– Nina Teicholz author, journalist, founder of the Nutrition Coalition

PART 1

THE THINGS I AM

To find yourself, think for yourself.

- Socrates

Chapter 1

There Is a Better Way

When things are going well we don't want them to change. Even when things are going just okay, we often don't want them to change. Change is rarely easy. Change is often painful.

When you're living your life, you don't want someone telling you that you will soon die.

December 7, 2009, the day I gave birth to Luna, the youngest of my three beautiful children, I'd gotten to my office at Salem Internal Medicine Practice, part of the Indiana University Health (IUH) system, around 6:30 a.m., a full day of patients ahead of me. But soon enough something was happening. I thought I might be going into labor, and I had never experienced that before: Noah and Ava were both induced. With Noah, I went in for a checkup at 37 weeks, the ob-gyn performed a non-stress test, saw that his heartbeat was dropping, and *That's it, let's get him out now*. With Ava, I was hospitalized at 29 weeks for preterm labor and made it to 37 weeks before being induced. I was the happiest pregnant person the first two times, up through the magic number of 37 weeks, then the kids got restless.

Pregnant with Luna, I was again the world's happiest person, and this time there was no rushing at the end. I hit nine months. Then, that morning in my office, I felt a tug. I announced to Tamara Hazbun, my colleague and close friend, "I think I'm going into labor." With the exception of my ob-gyn's office, there was no better place on Earth for this realization: Tamara was a family practice doctor. She had delivered hundreds of babies.

"Let me check you," she said, not missing a beat. We thought it was pretty funny for one friend to be examining the cervix of the other. For years after, Tamara liked to say, "I was the first one to touch Luna's head."

Her brief exam of me completed, Tamara announced, "Okay, you need to go to the hospital." It was an hour's drive from West Lafayette, Indiana, where my husband Brad and our kids and I lived, to IUH North, in Indianapolis. I planned to have the baby there because it's where Dr. Ball, the ob-gyn who had brought Noah and Ava into the world, practiced. If it ain't broke, right?

I was slightly stunned that Luna was ready. I was a novice at labor. I simply said, "Oh, okay."

"Call Brad," Tamara urged, amping things up. "Gotta get going."

And though I was in labor, and though there was still an hour's drive to Indy, and though I needed to let my husband know what was happening and have him come pick me up at the office and let Mom know to pick up the older kids from school, there was something else I needed to do, at least as important.

"I can't leave yet," I told Tamara.

Earlier that morning, tests results on Donald, one of my longest-standing patients, had come back, revealing acute leukemia. (I've changed the names of patients, to protect their privacy or that of their loved ones.) He had started feeling poorly a few weeks earlier and seemed to be getting worse fast. While I had hoped that Donald, in his early 60s, could survive for a while, the realist in me suspected he had just months to live, maybe weeks. He was not in good health to begin with. I wasn't going to give him an exact number – no one knows for sure – but he deserved the prognosis. And I wasn't leaving it to another doctor to give Donald the incredibly difficult news, though my being in labor was a pretty great excuse.

I called Donald at work. I told him he needed to come in. He said he couldn't get away just yet, though he knew it was important enough that I was the one calling, and troubling enough that I wouldn't tell him over the phone. He wanted an answer for why he'd been feeling so lousy but, then again, part of him didn't, terrified of the worst case. When I think back on it now, I wonder why he didn't insist that he truly couldn't leave work. Delay the face-to-face for a few hours, if not the anxiety.

In the meantime, I called Brad to come on over with the car and the overnight bag I'd packed. Tamara was shaking her head disapprovingly, knowing it was time to go, knowing I knew that. Brad arrived at the office, I was in labor – but still I wouldn't leave until Donald arrived. I didn't think I was taking a big risk. I had Tamara there. And as a mother and a doctor myself, I had a highly developed sense of risk.

About a half-hour later, Donald walked in. Behind the closed door of my office, I told him the horrible news. I stayed with him as long as I could, helping him to absorb it, though no one ever absorbs it. He stared blankly.

"I have to get better care for Angie," he said, the ultimate in practicality, selflessness, and love. Donald had been providing his wife Angie with round-the-clock care. She was morbidly obese, with uncontrolled diabetes, and neuropathy so bad she was in a wheelchair and almost blind. She herself was on death's door.

As the fact of his results sank in, Donald reeled. I did all I could to comfort him. Then the nurses came in and took over, and I ran out. Brad drove us, plus happy-dancing Luna inside me, seventy-five miles an hour to IUH North, where our third child, at 6 lbs. 5 oz., was born at 8:24 that evening.

Donald died in January, five and a half weeks later, before I returned to my practice from maternity leave.

~

I think of Donald's story as one of violent change. Yes, he was feeling bad before the test results were in, and he might well have suspected something could be really wrong, but the moment he learned of his death sentence, everything was different. Everything flipped. Going from one long held belief about yourself and the world to a very different one is jarring, at the least. In Donald's case and that of many people in his unfortunate situation, this change in belief is wrenching, horrible, involuntary. Wildly unwelcome.

But *any* significant change in belief is really hard, often painful. Even those you have agency over. It's not easy going from A to B. And it's *really* not easy going from A to Z.

Change. This book is about change. Specifically,

it is about the urgent need in America and the world – but especially America – to change what we eat. More generally, it's about the urgent need for us to challenge our *thinking* about food and health, thinking that is inadequate, misguided, and dangerously entrenched. I don't use the word "danger" lightly: The need for this change is, for so many, many people, a question of life and death.

Many of us believed – and still believe – falsehoods about food, nutrition, diet, and their effects on health. And we continue to think this way because a system was set up to preserve that way of thinking.

Not changing our thinking is literally killing us, millions of us. I know that sounds melodramatic. I'm sad to report that the facts bear it out. For decades, we've been told a story about diet and nutrition and health that was flat out wrong. There was precious little evidence for our national dietary recommendations, ones that were followed religiously for decades. These recommendations "sounded" right. At times, people in the know, well-meaning in their intentions, came to the wrong conclusion; other times, people in the know used outright deception and manipulation to make us believe something that turned out to be untrue. Once these recommendations settled in as the standard – the status quo – it became almost impossible to tell a different story.

Fortunately, there is another path we can take, a change we can make, that will help so many people live healthier, longer, better lives. I have been fortunate enough to be at the forefront of discoveries around this preferable path, and with a phenomenal team we have uncovered and laid bare the evidence of its benefits unlike anything that has come before. This path is scientific. The results are published and continually updated. Anyone can see what we've found. Unlike the "evidence" that supposedly supported the status quo dietary recommendations, our work is transparent, public, and thorough. Unfortunately, far too many in the medical and scientific establishments, for sometimes understandable reasons (e.g., it's tough to break from the pack; it takes time to see what's wrong) and for other times indefensible reasons, have moved very slowly or not at all in accepting this evidence. To do so would require ditching their thinking – status quo, factually insupportable, just plain wrong thinking.

Anything my colleagues and I do to help these evidence-based ideas gain momentum – and they are gaining momentum – means that some other idea is losing steam, and its believers will resist the change. My work has focused on nutrition and obesity, nutrition and diabetes. There has been pushback, but it's crucial to communicate the notion that (a) *the obesity epidemic can be conquered* and (b) *type 2 diabetes can be reversed* – not just managed.[1] Before fairly recently, no one entertained the concept of reversal. Thanks in part to social media, which enables new voices to be heard, that momentum can change quickly.

As promising as it is to have a new path, making the change will not be easy. It will be hard, very hard. But it is necessary. Because the status quo is killing us. Just as important, the status quo has been diminishing hope for so many people who are suffering right now who shouldn't have to. When there's no hope that real

---

[1] Reversal of diabetes means that blood sugar drops to normal levels without medication (except possibly metformin).

change can happen, it doesn't. Simple as that. My wish is that when you get to the end of this book, I will have persuaded you of the need to make this change, and of the need to find and work with healthcare practitioners who understand it too. If that happens, then I am certain you will be happy about it, even transformed.

There is one change I know is not possible: my being around when you get to the end of this book. I will not. Like my patient Donald, one moment I was living my life, the next someone was giving me my own death sentence. That happened the last day of June, 2017, when I was 45. Noah was 14, Ava was 12, and Luna was 7. Because I am a doctor, a researcher, a mom, a wife, a daughter, a sister, a friend, a fighter, I did everything I could to change the outcome. Of course I did. I told myself, in one of countless delusional moments, *I just want eleven years*. Not so I would make it to 56 years old (a rather arbitrary number), but because by then, Luna would be 18 and I would have just enough time to help her move into her freshman dorm at college.

I fought as much as I could and staved off death for a while – until I couldn't. Most people with my diagnosis are gone in a few years. When you read this book, I will be dead, from non-smoking lung cancer.

The American healthcare system is amazing in many ways, but it could be far, far better in so many important ways, and these are not pipe dreams I'm talking about. These are real possibilities. Status quo thinking is not just holding back better health outcomes for the people I mostly worked with for the last 10 years – those suffering from obesity, or type 2 diabetes (T2D), or both – but it impacts other areas of health care, including the delivery of medical services. Status quo thinking is a major reason why inequities are with us, and growing worse, in 21st century American health care.

Through my firsthand experience, I want to show why everyone in America and beyond should care about what's going on. This is not just about my patients. This is about patients all over. What you don't know *can* hurt you. *Is* hurting you.

This is my story, and it's your story, too.

I urge you to hear what my colleagues and I discovered, as well as the findings of the brilliant scientists and researchers who came before us and alongside us and right this very minute, so that you may live a longer, healthier, better life than the one you are experiencing right now.

This book is about a willingness to change our thinking and not get stuck in the status quo, particularly when it's harming us. Taking *control* over change. This may sound odd coming from someone who is no longer around as you read these words, but as much as this book is about status quo thinking and changing it, it is also about hope. Because if we can't have hope that there's a better way out there, when we know for sure that there's something very wrong with the current state of things, then how do we go on?

There is a better way.

~   ~   ~

Chapter 2

Pivots

The best health care is a combination of medical fact, competent execution, and human feeling. It requires the expertise of the doctor or medical professional, but also the active engagement and choice of the patient. In a very real sense, you could say that great health care is all about trust – who you trust, and why.

What I advocate in this book comes from following the science. But my years of experience – as physician, as head of an obesity clinic, as lead investigator in a paradigm-busting nutrition study, and as medical director for a telemedicine company focused on reversing (not managing; *reversing*) type 2 diabetes – have taught me that what is vital for success is the human element, the trust, and the level at which patient and doctor understand each other.

Since I'm asking you to make a leap in your thinking, perhaps even to renounce ideas you believe or have been told to believe for decades, it's only fair that you first understand the person who's suggesting that leap. And since this is the one shot I'll get at talking directly to you (aside from various videos of me that you can find on the internet), I hope the story of my own personal, intellectual, and scientific journey explains how I became such an enemy of the status quo in medicine. I hope my story engenders your trust.

~

I'm the only person I know of who disappointed her parents when she announced she wanted to be a doctor.

I didn't grow up thinking I would be one. At no point in my childhood did the thought cross my mind. My parents were both academics – John, my dad, an associate professor of finance at Northern Illinois University in DeKalb, and Ellen, my mom, with a position in survey research at NIU's Center for Governmental Studies. It was an unwritten idea in our family that my sister and I would choose fields we liked and become professors in them. Night follows day.

But after four years in college, then time in grad school to get a master's in exercise physiology, I had my *Aha!* moment and realized that medicine was the field I liked best and, maybe more importantly, the one that made me angriest. I wanted – *needed* – to practice my discipline, not teach it. I dreaded the call announcing my decision.

"What? Are you kidding?" my parents said, each in their own ways.

It meant staying an extra year in grad school to take all the undergraduate classes I never took that were pre-reqs for medical school. It meant turning down the assistantship in exercise physiology that Purdue University had just offered me on the road to a PhD.

Now I knew what I was going to do with my life, at least professionally. I was going to be a cardiologist. For sure.

~

With a mom and dad both in academics, research was the heart and soul of my family. Though I would ultimately diverge from the path they thought I was on, it took a while, along with a moment of outrage (okay, more than one), for me to move to outright, action-oriented doctoring. And since outrage and passion have fueled me as much as anything, and helped uncover the important discoveries that my colleagues and I ultimately made, I think it's worth explaining who got me so royally angry, and how.

While getting my master's degree in exercise physiology with Dr. Dale Brown as my thesis chair, I had yet to be bitten by the doctor bug. I was glad to be getting another degree, and to know I had a career waiting in a field that excited me. (My thesis set out to answer the question, which style of exercise on the Stairmaster – taking lots of smaller steps versus fewer and bigger strides – burned more calories. The winner? Fewer and bigger.) Plus, Brad, who I met and began dating freshman year, and I were now engaged, and he had one more year to get his bachelor's in public health.

But that period in my life illuminated some things I hadn't realized before. First was the revelation that I lived in a bubble. One married friend, from a working-class background, with a husband who had a steady job at an automobile plant, was the first in her family to go to college, getting a bachelor's in environmental sciences. I so admired that she was doing something that practically no one in her circle had done before. Another friend, who referred to himself as a Trailer Park Kid, had upset his family by pursuing a PhD; they wanted him just to get a job already. That wasn't uncommon. Lots of my classmates and college friends were the first in their families to get formal education past high school. Several who were doing graduate work expressed dismay at the pressure they felt to quit and get a "real job." One of them said to me – without bitterness, just to make a point – "Not everyone comes from a family where both parents are professors."

I understood how fortunate I was.

My parents were thrilled, of course, by my graduate school journey. I felt no conflict about spending another year or two in school. We weren't affluent but comfortably middle-class, and never had to worry about paying the monthly bills or having enough medical insurance, as friends sometimes agonized over. One friend at Illinois State was a mom of two who had just gone through a nasty divorce. My mother and my sister Jenna came down from DeKalb, and the three of us went Christmas shopping for my friend and her kids, because Mom was concerned that they wouldn't have gifts. Mom always led by example.

~

Then I learned something else, and everything changed.

Back when I was a college senior I had taken a job at a local hospital as an exercise physiologist in the cardiac rehab department, with three rotating responsibilities: monitoring arrhythmias in the "cath" (for catheter) lab, overseeing stress tests, and helping patients with their rehab.

In my second year on the job – during my first year of grad school – I was putting in a lot more hours because I had fewer hours in the classroom. I was excited about the path I was on. I had just been accepted by Purdue for a PhD, including an assistantship, in exercise physiology.

I knew my work provided meaningful value to our cardiac patients. One of my favorites, a man named Ken who had experienced both coronary artery disease and heart failure, was always so appreciative of the hands-on work I did with him. I helped increase stamina and build strength in his heart muscle by pushing him on, carefully monitoring his treadmill exercises. The point was to decrease risk factors, one of which is sedentary behavior. As with most people, Ken responded well to encouragement, physical touch, smiles. Wow, who could have predicted that? For Ken and his wife Carrie, also a cardiac patient, and everyone else who came through, I did whatever I could to make them feel better and improve their situation. Ken and Carrie were both obese, and both committed to exercising more. The one real change they made in their diet, a change I encouraged, was to eat less high-fat food.

When I was on duty in the cath lab, the place patients came when they had chest pain that appeared cardiac in origin, my role was to follow their EKG "tracings" and call out if there was any sign of arrhythmia, or abnormal heartbeat. Often I worked with a cardiologist I'll call Dr. Mark Conklin. Even on his best day, there is no way to describe Dr. Conklin as anything but a total pompous ass.

Because I was neither a doctor nor a registered nurse, to Dr. Conklin I was merely an extra, one of many faceless individuals on his "pay no mind" list. More than just lacking interest in my existence, he had zero respect for me and what I did in my job that might help him in his. The only exchanges we had, much like the exchanges he had with seemingly everyone else at the hospital who was not a doctor or an RN (though he had his share of dismissive exchanges with nurses, too, because, after all, they weren't doctors, and generally not men), consisted of him yelling at me or us, constantly, about our ineptitude and worthlessness.

On one particular day in the lab, I watched the screens, knowing I needed to alert Dr. Conklin in the event of significant arrhythmias. I say "significant" because single "abnormal" heartbeats happen all the time, to people with perfectly good hearts. You have them, I have them, everyone has them. An arrhythmia is significant only when there are multiple off-rhythm beats strung together. To point out every time a single abnormal beat occurs, when it's followed immediately by an extended return to normalcy, is pointless.

I knew how busy the doctors were, and that I had a certain amount of discretion about when to alert the staff about a potential situation. One abnormal beat did not make a situation.

On this day, one of the patients registered a single abnormal beat, then returned immediately to normal. But Dr. Conklin happened to look at the monitor exactly during that sequence, and when I didn't say anything to him, he did what he always did: He screamed. In this instance, at me.

My response? I did not talk back. But from that moment on, I decided to notify Dr. Conklin and the entire lab of every single abnormal beat that registered. *EVERY ONE.* I called out, sometimes in intervals of every few seconds, "Arrhythmia! . . . Arrhythmia! . . .

Arrhythmia!" I was going to be an ass right back to Dr. Conklin because I was so mad at how he treated me (and others), at how certain he was that I had no idea what I was doing, and that his judgment was infallible and mine was, well, non-existent.

I followed my plan for about five minutes before Dr. Conklin blew up at me again, this time for causing such a disturbance. In front of everyone, he demeaned and demoralized me.

And in that moment, my career path changed forever. *You know what?* I told myself. *They're never going to listen to you.*

I was so mad.

Anger is a persuasive emotion. It can be destructive as hell. And it can be such a powerful motivator. It can drive innovation, creativity, and bold decisions.

Bold decision, here I come.

Dr. Conklin, a cardiologist, possessed a limited, important type of knowledge and expertise, but he never got what the phrase "health care" truly meant. To him, it was a transaction, nothing more. And he was a complete ass.

Yet he was the one everybody called Doctor.

By the time he had spent the last of his vitriol on me for that day's rant, something had come over me, then and there. I realized I was not going to be an exercise physiologist, much as I loved the field and thought it was of vital importance to use exercise to help patients suffering from chronic diseases, especially heart and lung. I would still integrate its principles into whatever health care I ultimately provided patients.

No, I was on a new path.

I was going to go to medical school.

I was going to be a doctor. More than that, I was going to be a cardiologist.

I was going to say no to the PhD offer at Purdue. I really didn't look forward to that phone call with my parents.

But I felt that the only way to earn respect in the medical field and have people truly listen to what I had to say, whether it was about exercise or anything else that I had researched for myself and used to positive effect on actual people, was to do it as a doctor.

If you can't beat 'em – right?

~

Whenever I finally did become a doctor, it was going to be hard-earned: I had gotten a master's degree, then a job, and only *then* was I bitten by the doctor bug. Since DO (Doctor of Osteopathic Medicine) schools were known to value non-traditional students, and embrace those with real-life experience in health care and working with patients, I thought, *That's where I belong. That's me.* I started at Des Moines University in 1998.

The way it worked at that school: you were unlikely to do your third and fourth years there because the city of Des Moines wasn't big enough to handle all the medical students who needed slots for clinical rotations. For my third year of medical school, I went to St. John's Westlake Hospital, just outside of Cleveland.

My education had barely begun.

~

You can stay on a well-worn path or veer off it, unsure if there's a better one. You can keep to a belief, maybe even a somewhat damaging belief, and stick with it because you don't want to look silly or stupid by abandoning an idea that you have spent so much time following and maybe even championing; you may hold on because you're too scared to see what a different belief might lead to. Maybe you stick with it simply because everyone else is, too, including storied institutions and wealthy organizations and supposedly esteemed people.

Or you can dig deep, deeper, to see for yourself if this cherished belief might be something other than true. One of the best personal examples of digging deeper, going beyond shallow knowledge, is also one of the most memorable patient encounters I ever had. It involved a cardiologist named Dr. Atul Hulyalkar whom I assisted on rotation at St. John's.

One day we were called to the Intensive Care Unit (ICU) because of a "code": A "code blue," usually shortened to "code," is announced throughout the hospital when a patient needs immediate attention for an irregular heart rhythm or respiratory distress. There is a rush by doctors, nurses, and respiratory therapists to the patient's room. In this case, the patient's blood pressure was crashing. When I arrived, the ICU specialists were already there, surrounding the patient, about to give her a "pressor": medication to increase her blood pressure by constricting the vessels, via intravenous (IV).

Dr. Hulyalkar quickly evaluated the situation and directed the nurse, "Give her a beta blocker."

We all looked at him. He had to be mistaken.

"No, I'm not doing that," the nurse said, resolutely. The patient's blood pressure was crashing – and the doctor wanted to give her a medication that *lowers* blood pressure? Still, the nurse, knowing her responsibility, filled the syringe with the beta blocker.

Dr. Hulyaklar instructed her again to administer the medication.

"You'll kill her!" said the nurse.

This was dramatic stuff. You didn't talk back to doctors like that. You certainly didn't refuse to carry out their orders.

Dr. Hulyaklar turned to the ICU doctor and instructed him to administer the medicine. He too refused. "No way," he said.

A shouting match ensued – but time was slipping away and finally Dr. Hulyalkar shook his head, furious, and hollered, "Give me the syringe!" Reluctantly, the nurse handed it to him. I will never forget the gasps when he jammed the syringe into the IV running into the woman's arm.

Almost instantly her blood pressure rose.

The whole exchange took no more than thirty seconds, tops, though it seemed operatic in the back and forth.

Dr. Hulyalkar explained to everyone assembled what had been going on: The patient was suffering from hypertrophic cardiomyopathy, meaning the blood pressure was dropping because the heart was constricting, cutting off the arterial supply to the heart. By giving her blood pressure medication, the doctor was relaxing the heart enough to allow blood flow again.

You need to understand everything that goes into the system to understand that. You need to know the rules as well as the exceptions to the rules to make a counterintuitive call like that, particularly under pressure, when it's life and death. No one else in that room had all that knowledge but the top doctor. Yet everyone was willing to defy him – understandably – though their understanding was inferior to his.

I'm pretty sure that everyone standing around the patient remembers that moment to this day. I've often wondered if the nurse and the ICU head who defied Dr. Hulyalkar both thought, *Well, there goes my career.* Once the tension had eased, I remember thinking, *You are my hero! Will I ever be able to own a situation like that?* I was determined that someday *I* would have deep enough knowledge and understanding to perform like Dr. Hulyalkar and save a life. And he had not merely saved a life, but he then taught the gathered medical staff how he knew to do what he had done. All of us there knew that the patient's symptoms – shortness of breath, chest pain, edema – could be signs of decompensating hypertrophic cardiomyopathy, and some there even knew she had been diagnosed with it. They just didn't understand it, really. Everyone there, except for me, had been caring for the patient the past couple days. Dr. Hulyalkar pointed out to us that, in panicked moments, it is critical to remember *everything* you know, and then make a decision based on that, *whatever it might be.* To practice "cookbook medicine" – medical decisions that narrowly follow the book, and don't allow for the aberrations that inevitably happen in real life – could be deadly. To get the blood pressure up, we actually needed to give medicine that relaxed rather than constricted. I knew then that cookbook medicine was not for me.

After we walked out, Dr. Hulyalkar sat me down in a nearby conference room and explained things further. He was such a busy man yet he gave me time because he could see I was genuinely interested to know more.

"You can't fix things unless you understand them," he said simply. "You can't always just take things at face value, what seems the logical step. You must first have a genuine understanding of the physiology and chemistry to make the best choice."

I knew what he was saying was true in a general sense. I didn't realize just how true it would be for the specific medical path I would embark on in the years to come.

~

I wanted to become a doctor partly because I like people, I like helping them, and I like seeing them transformed by things I've encouraged them to do.

But I'm also obsessed with the science behind what we do, not just its clinical application. I love knowing *how* things work. Maybe I got that from my dad, whose first career was as an engineer. When I was 11, I created a Rube Goldberg machine that started in my bedroom, where I would pull on a string when I woke up in the morning. The string connected to other strings and wires leading to the bathroom down the hall, where a hammer would be released, smash the toothpaste tube and – in a perfect world – the toothpaste would squirt onto my toothbrush. I titled it "THE MARVOLIS INVENTION of SARAH DRAN." It never worked.

No matter. My enthusiasm did not wane. I think this little misadventure foretold my adult striving to find links, what *really* leads to what, and to keep at it, to keep working things over.

My appetite for the way things connect in medicine was voracious. I always wanted to understand the true, deep part, not just, *If Person A has Condition A, then give them Medicine A.* Because – wait – does that always make the most sense? Does it even make the most sense half the time? Could Medicine B be just as good, with fewer side effects? What about no medicine at all? Is Condition A really all that's going on? So much health care is by the book (Problem #1) and the book isn't always right to begin with (Problem #2).

The issues caused by these two problems are not always, or even most of the time, the fault of doctors. The system encourages a rote approach. The culture encourages it. And in so many ways, this approach is failing us, producing disastrous results.

A lot of my own thinking about health was inspired by the influence of Dr. Hulyalkar and other creative, restless thinkers I've been privileged to work with over the years.

Restlessness. Impatience. Dissatisfaction. Anger. These can be healthy, productive emotional states and mindsets. Big things rarely get accomplished without them. Keepers of the status quo certainly don't appreciate them. But speaking up, standing up, talking back – yelling! – can be tough, particularly for women. Yet we have to do it. I think of the time when my husband Brad and I had just moved from Cleveland to Indianapolis, where I had a residency in internal medicine at St. Vincent's. When I walked into the

21

hospital on my first day of work, I was more nervous than usual because I was seven months pregnant, my first. Fortunately, I'd been assured that St. Vincent's was very family-friendly when it came to its staff. I got introduced to my new colleagues. They were all nice and reassuring, with one caveat.

"You'll be fine," said one of the young doctors, "as long as you don't match with Dr. Byron." A second person agreed. A third nodded.

I probably don't have to tell you who I got matched with.

As I walked around during my rotation with Dr. William Byron, the hospital's chief of critical care, he was brutal in his manner and demands. He expected you to read and fully understand pages of research every night, all based on a question he had asked of you earlier that day. They were pulmonary critical care questions – this one on ventilator management, that one on outpatient management. It was a practice I'd been through as a medical student, but now Dr. Byron pushed me or whatever young doctor he had with him.

Oh, my god, I thought, *I'm going to die from the amount of work, the pressure, the exhaustion. I'm extremely pregnant. How am I going to succeed?*

The second week, a patient in the hospital coded. Dr. Byron and I wound up on the same floor. At the patient's bedside, Dr. Byron barked, "Hallberg, intubate!"

Holy crap. I had never intubated anybody.

Yet here we were mid-code, and he was telling me to intubate this poor guy. I failed in my first attempt. I failed in my second attempt. I was trying again when Dr. Byron yelled, "*Goddamnit, Hallberg!*" and began swearing at my ineptitude. I tried to tune out the cursing as I kept on with my attempt to intubate the patient.

Finally, as his swearing continued, I snapped my head up at him and, with building volume, exploded, "You are not helping me . . . *I have to concentrate . . . SHUT UP!*"

But for the beeping machines in the room there was total silence. Nobody there could believe I had just yelled at the chief of critical care. It just came out. With the combination of frustration, pressure, unnecessary screaming and venom from him, I did exactly what needed to be done in the moment. I screamed right back and told him to shut up.

Then I intubated the patient successfully.

The exchange altered my relationship with Dr. Byron. It was an indelible moment in my professional life. He and I became almost friends – as much as you can be friends in a fundamentally mentor-student relationship. I did multiple rotations with him, learning so much each time. Many of my most important and memorable adventures in the ICU were either with him or employing knowledge I had gained from him. I sometimes think about all I wouldn't have learned if I had swallowed that "Shut Up!" And how talking back led to my arguments with the status quo.

~

As a doctor, there were other forks in my road, and these had to do as much with the How behind medicine as the What and Why. I don't think you can fully solve or improve things without a genuinely humane approach. The How isn't some "add-on"; it can deeply, objectively

23

affect the What and the Why. How to behave. How to command. How to speak.

I had logged enough experiences with doctors who couldn't or wouldn't communicate with others – not just with patients, their most important audience, but also with colleagues, assistants, families of patients, etc. There was the incident with Dr. Conklin and the "abnormal" heart beat that led to my pivot to medicine. Another notable incident occurred after I made that decision and was spending a year studying for the medical school entrance exam – the MCAT. At the time I worked in another cardiac rehab unit. Once again I found myself working with another ass of a doctor. He was remarkably similar to Dr. Conklin in how he saw zero value in anyone who was not a doctor. Everyone else was background noise. So Dr. Conklin was not the only pompous one out there, as I would discover and rediscover over the course of my career.

But I don't regret enduring both of them because they taught me something of great value: the importance of communication.

I hope it's not immodest to say, but one of my earliest realizations about myself had been that I was a good communicator. My communication skill may have been cultivated by growing up in a household with a generally poor communicator, my dad, who was probably on the Asperger's spectrum, which wasn't identified when he was young (no one, in his day, was being identified like that). Painful as it was to experience this friction, it was a gift in its way. You really work to communicate with someone who's bad at it. And I became a more *creative* communicator because of it.

Creative communication starts, naturally, with listening, a skill that the average doctor is legendarily bad at because (a) patients come to him or her precisely to avail themselves of his or her knowledge and skills, and (b) doctors are told for so many years that they're the smartest person in the room. To me, creative communication means letting the patient tell you, the doctor, his or her story; and for you, the doctor, to talk to the patient in the way that's most comfortable for him or her. One study showed that doctors interrupt their patients after an average of eleven seconds. Can we even call that communication?

To be the most effective doctor possible, doesn't it make sense to talk with different patients differently, in the same way that you would prescribe different dosages of medications, depending on the type and severity of the patient's condition?

Creative communication merely means not trying to communicate the same way with everyone. It's meeting patients where they are, where they feel most comfortable and where they will be most receptive. Sometimes you talk faster, sometimes slower. Your analogies should be different. For some, you get out a pen and paper and diagram what's going on.

You might communicate differently with a patient who is in your office alone versus one who brings a family member to listen and advocate; with a patient whose English is halting versus one who is fluent; with a patient who is a Type A personality versus one who seems indecisive or insecure; with a patient who has a long history of always putting the needs of loved ones before her own versus a patient who is decidedly not that; with a patient who is really involved in his or her own health versus one who just wants to get the hell out of there.

Because if you don't alter your style? You'll get through to only a small subset of people for whom your particular communication style works. You'll be ineffective with others. Some people you'll confuse. Some you'll insult.

To communicate well, it also helps to express sympathy; if it's genuine, that's so much better. That's a gift if you sometimes have to tell people awful stuff. It probably sounds depressing and terrifying to have one of your occupational responsibilities be delivering bad news – even the worst news – to people. For me, it was the opposite. I told myself: *In the most terrible moment, Sarah, you're capable of giving them what many others can't. Explain everything plainly, listen, answer questions, and remember:* **touch***. Touching is so important in this situation, even for the most standoffish patients. When absorbing bad news, people need human touch. Hold their hands, drape your arm over their shoulders, hug them while they cry. Maybe you'll cry with them. Each person is different, but be willing to touch or hold them while they absorb and grieve. That's the most important thing you can do, initially. A genuine human act of connection.*

I learned always to think about the patients and how they were feeling at that very minute. No matter what kind of day I was having, the patient deserved 100% empathy, 100% attention.

While I was a resident at St. Vincent's, there were many shifts when it was a dozen interns (rookie residents) and me. Often, when they were dealing with a dire situation, and had to share a piece of tragic information with a patient or their loved ones, the interns would come get me. They wanted nothing to do with it. I was the Grim Reaper, though as a generally buoyant, wide-eyed, 5'4½" optimist, I don't know that I looked the part. Which might, of course, have helped. "Okay, I'll talk to them," I told my colleagues who couldn't. And so I was often the designated dispenser of difficult news; I delivered verdicts as humanely as I could. When I was doing it for other doctors, it was usually the first time I was meeting the patient or the family or other loved ones. I don't know if it made things worse or better (or neither) for them that this stranger was giving them the dreaded news. It wasn't that the intern knew them so much better than I did, but certainly she or he had at least interacted with them for a few days, before the sickening clarity about the patient's condition was confirmed.

Of course, most of the news I delivered touched on death. Confronted it, if in a gentle way.

We really don't know if he's going to make it.

We think you should go into the room to be with her.

Sit with her. And then when you're ready, let's call the family in. We can stay together until they all get here. I'm right here with you.

How you are may be just as important as *What* you know. Both are needed to help your patients and to advocate for the best possible treatment and outcome.

~   ~   ~

Chapter 3

Motherhood and Hope

The eighth day of October 2002, everything turned upside down for me.

Again. Forever.

For the first time in years, I questioned what kind of doctor I wanted to be.

That was the day I became a mother.

It was as abrupt as the day I went from wanting to be an exercise physiologist to wanting to be a doctor. The moment I first held Noah was the moment I gave up cardiology. I went into the hospital to give birth, and came out utterly in love with this new creature, and just as utterly unsure of what came next in my career. Suddenly, all I thought about cardiology was how it would require me to spend almost three years finishing my internal medicine residency, then *another* three years in an intense cardiology fellowship, mostly away from him – never mind the promises of how family-friendly my new employer was supposed to be.

When my eight weeks of maternity leave ended, I was even more sure that a major change was necessary. Returning to work was horrible. On those occasions where I had to be at the hospital overnight and into the next day – those brutal, insane 32-hour shifts from 7 in the morning until 3 the following afternoon – the crying started after about 24 hours. Standing there as the attending doctor did rounds, I would bawl my eyes out, part blinding exhaustion, part missing Noah so crazy hard.

I was beyond tired all the time. My exhaustion led me to investigate how I might work less hard and be more available to Noah. *Maybe I should be a vein specialist*, I thought. I knew that physicians were being hired to perform a relatively routine laser procedure to remove spider veins and varicose veins, and were paid well to do so.

Yes! I would forego my cardiology fellowship, and I'd be practicing in just over two years. I'd have a job at a clinic helping women (mostly) and men get rid of unsightly veins. As medicine goes, that was an easy life.

But was "easy" what I wanted?

Sure, I'll do that, a job with actual normal hours! No working nights! No 30-hour shifts! More time with the baby!

No.

I couldn't work just on leg veins. Yes, I wanted to find a way to be much more with Noah, but I didn't want easy. I knew I would be bored. Also, when I had been through a rotation at a vein clinic, it seemed as if everyone who walked in was getting the laser procedure. You don't want a specialist who thinks *everyone* needs that treatment, so I wasn't feeling great about that. I was determined to change my circumstances as a doctor for my new circumstances as a mom, yet I just couldn't do that. If I sound as if I'm dissing doctors who do opt for that specialty and that life, I'm not: It just wasn't for me.

There had to be a third way. There was.

I would be a doctor doctor. Primary care, for adults. It would still mean time away from Noah – I would have to do two more years of my internal medicine residency, and the occasional long night was unavoidable. But my overall career arc would not be nearly as soul-crushing as cardiology. I would be a doctor, but one who might have a life.

That was the new plan. Another pivot.

~

In my third and final year of residency, while very pregnant with Ava, my second child, I had my single most important patient experience. To this day, for all the patient moments in my career, this one still has not been topped in how deeply it affected me and the way I thought and practiced.

I was on for the overnight shift in the ICU when my fellow resident, finishing his shift, sat with me to share patient developments. He told me that a woman had been admitted with a suspected urinary tract infection (UTI) but was experiencing "a lot more pain and her condition seems more complicated." My colleague continued: "She doesn't seem completely stable and she's having classic symptoms of pyelo." Pyelonephritis is inflammation of the kidney that can accompany a certain type of urinary tract infection. "For now, we're treating it like a UTI."

It was now just me in the ICU. I went to look in on the patient early in my shift. The woman was awake, and looked younger than her listed age of 46. She was thin, though her belly was slightly distended. She was groggy – not surprising because of the pain medicine she'd been put on, along with antibiotics. Her husband sat bedside. He looked defeated.

I walked into the room to introduce myself since I would be there all night. He looked at me with the saddest eyes.

"Well, this has been the worst day of our lives," he said.

"Please tell me what you mean," I said.

"My wife has a condition called neurofibromatosis," he said.

With this disease, people develop tumors (fibroma) on nerves (neuro), which can pop up anywhere and cause problems. Sometimes the tumors are visible, but usually they're internal, so observers don't know their true nature. The pain, I had learned, can be excruciating. There is no cure. There really is no treatment either.

The husband told me that his wife had developed a tumor high on her cervical spine. It had been discovered four months before. The two of them had been going from one neurosurgeon to another, soliciting opinions. One after the other had told them it was inoperable – removal would cause paralysis. But so, ultimately, would doing nothing.

Their last ditch, "Hail Mary" appointment with yet another neurosurgeon had happened earlier that day. As with the others, the doctor soberly told both of them that nothing could be done about the tumor. It would continue to grow until it paralyzed her from the neck down, probably within months.

Now, as the patient's husband finished pouring out the sad details of their story to me, he said, "This just seems like a fitting ending for the day. She finally lost hope."

The last four words hit me with such visceral power, I blurted, "Oh my god" – but any further conversation, at least for the moment, was interrupted because she was crashing: She was quickly "decompensating" – functionally deteriorating – though still initially awake.

I ushered the husband out of the room. As the interns, nurses, and I tended to her, I wanted her sent to the CT scanner to figure out what was happening, but she needed to be stabilized first or she wouldn't survive transport. The on-call physician agreed when the intern called her. And there was another problem: It was proving extremely difficult to intubate the woman, because of another manifestation of her condition. Some of her tumors had caused nerve irritation in her neck, causing torticollis, a condition where the neck has been tilted to the side for so long, it deforms and can't be straightened. We paralyzed her airway – typical for intubation but particularly so when there's torticollis – yet we still struggled. She had the smallest airway I'd ever worked on so we used a pediatric tube. By now, I was a whiz at intubation, a far cry from that first, charged experience with Dr. Byron, yet I couldn't get the tube in. We called for anesthesia while the interns continued to "bag" the patient (manually pumping air into her lungs). I decided to let two of the interns try to intubate the patient. Maybe I was having a bad night. It happens.

At some point during the scramble, the chief of the unit walked in. It was unusual for him to be there at that time. He had come to check on someone else, but because of the commotion, he stopped by the woman's bed. Even he had difficulty intubating her – but he finally succeeded.

Through the woman's IV, I put her on pressors, the medication used to keep blood pressure up, while also watching her heart rhythm on the monitor. Still good. But her belly was distending more. It was now clear that she had what's called a "surgical abdomen," meaning something was happening that could be resolved only by going into the abdomen and looking. The signs for this can be extreme bloating, profuse and consistent rectal bleeding, fever, and intense belly pain. Something catastrophic was happening but we didn't know what. I yelled for the intern to get the surgeon on the phone.

The patient's belly was getting worse. She was on pressors. She was, in a word, on life support. We had to figure out what was going on. She was stable enough now to go for a CT, which I knew was imperative. While the surgeon was being called by the intern, a nurse went to get the woman's husband.

When he got to the ICU room, I motioned for him to come in. He looked at his wife and began to weep.

"This may be for the best," he said, through tears. "How can you live without hope?"

Now I started crying.

"I don't want her to go to surgery," he said. "She wouldn't want this. None of this."

She crashed again and needed to be coded. Another flurry of activity began – but the husband asked us not to proceed.

She died.

It was all so quick.

It was one of my most tortuous nights ever, as a doctor and as a human being.

A woman who had been admitted just hours before with complications from what appeared to be a UTI was now dead.

Because it wasn't a UTI. It wasn't even serious complications from a UTI. As the autopsy would reveal, she had another new tumor – not the one she had been looking to have surgically removed. It was a tumor not externally visible when she was admitted. It had grown through her mesenteric artery, the big vessel that supplies blood to the gut. She was hemorrhaging from there, which explained her rapidly distending belly.

Even had we operated successfully, what would we be saving her *for*? To awaken to the prognosis that she had only a couple months until she was paralyzed? That other horrible tumors might be taking over? Once she had that meeting with the surgeon earlier that day, she was sapped of hope, one of the most important elements for survival. She told her husband she couldn't live without hope.

And so she didn't.

Her husband was right. This was the "best" way for it to end.

I have thought about that night, that harrowing experience, countless times over the years. I have thought about it for my many patients who were made to feel hopeless because their conditions have been harmed – often even *caused* – by status quo thinking. They were made to feel as if the problem was mostly or exclusively them rather than, in large part, the recommendations they had been given all their lives. I have thought about that night even more in the years since my own diagnosis.

Can any of us live without hope?

~

No. That's my answer to that question. I believe that no one can live without hope. The ability to stay hopeful seems one of the common threads for people who survive suffering. There are those who are hopeful who don't make it, of course – I'm betting I'm one of those – or whose outcome is otherwise not what they had, well, hoped for. Without hope, though, things become so much more difficult, for the present and the future.

When it comes to chronic disease, physicians and other healthcare providers have always had to walk the line between giving too much hope – false hope – and enabling enough of it, so people can continue to enjoy the time they have. But here's the thing: hope is not doled out equally in our healthcare system. If you're suffering from chronic disease, to maintain hope you must possess, among other things, a certain amount of confidence in the system charged with caring for you.

~   ~   ~

Chapter 4

Fed Up

On October 13, 2004, Ava was born at St. Vincent's.

As with Noah, I took my eight-week maternity leave, which would prolong the time before I finished my residency and moved on. But that was fine with me: clearly I was on the "delayed plan" to becoming a full-fledged doctor. And I had finally arrived at a point in my training where things weren't quite so grueling. The emotions of missing my new newborn, of missing both my children, were still intense. But the load would soon be lightened once we moved to West Lafayette, and I began work at Indiana University Health (IUH) Arnett Clinic in Lafayette.

As a primary care doctor – in my case, an internist for adult patients – you deal with everything and anything. Sinus infections, viral GI bugs, sleep problems, diabetes. People having heart attacks staggered in. So many people came in with depression and other mental/psychiatric issues, expecting that I was the one who might solve their problem. I was surprised that so much of the illness I saw was mental and emotional rather than simply physical.

I was lucky to work with Joni Anderson, a reliable and energetic medical assistant, by my side soon after I started at IUH. She was great at what she did and we came to rely on each other.

But there was a troubling issue, something systemic, going on with my practice.

The primary care system I was boxed into – as so many doctors had to practice it, and so many patients had to endure it – was miserable, ineffective, demeaning, shortsighted. Healthcare systems are maddeningly bureaucratic. Even individual visits between patient and doctor could be impersonal and inadequate. After all the years of classwork and research and training and grand rounds and residencies and specialized residencies and fellowships, all we were really trained and encouraged to do was one simple task:

Prescribe drugs.

That's it.

When I was on weekend call, some days I would get 20 requests from patients calling for an antibiotic. They did it because they had been conditioned to get these medications. They had come to expect that that was the answer, probably the only answer.

"I have a stuffy nose."

"How long?"

"Since yesterday. I need antibiotics."

Or: "I have pressure in my ear and my doctor always gives me antibiotics for it."

Patients had come to see doctors more and more as simply the people who prescribe drugs. I didn't blame the patients. Their expectations were driven by how easily their doctors, some of whom were my professional partners, would cave. I announced that I was not going to play that game.

"I am not sending in antibiotics on call anymore," I informed my staff, my colleagues, and anyone who would listen. "If the patient is sick enough to need an antibiotic, then they first need to be seen by someone."

The medical inappropriateness of overprescribing, especially over the phone, was insane. After all, what if the patient was worse than initially thought and had, say, pneumonia? Studies show that for respiratory tract infections (the impetus for a significant percentage of my on-call requests), more than 90% of prescriptions are unnecessary; most such infections are viral, so antibiotics won't help the problem. More than 90%! But the incentives placed on doctors screwed everything up. Because doctors grew so worried about undertreating and perhaps being charged with malpractice, the way they practiced medicine changed, as did the quality of care that patients received.

When I was on call, handling calls from patients, most of whom were not mine, I now often responded to their wish for a prescription – *I want medication*! – by telling them, "First you have to be seen by urgent care," and I could just hear the air go out of them. They weren't used to that answer. It's not what they expected. I would tell them, "Let's set up a time for you to come into your primary care physician's office tomorrow." *No, let's not*!

I pissed off lots of patients. A couple of them even filed complaints because they did not receive an antibiotic prescription with just a phone call.

But patients couldn't legitimately complain about my behavior: Medically, it was the right thing to do. It's estimated that one-third to one-half of *all* antibiotic prescriptions are unnecessary and may lead to complications.

To Brad and our friends, I started referring to my job as "legal drug dealer." My schedule, like that of so many internists and primary care doctors all over the country, allowed me no time to focus on preventive care. Once upon a time I had been so excited about helping people get healthy, or at least get less sick, by teaching them what I knew about the benefits of exercise and, by the way, healthy eating and proper sleep and other lifestyle changes. And true, I *did* initiate preventive measures for my patients, such as ordering colonoscopies, cholesterol and diabetes screening, and mammograms and breast MRIs in high-risk women.

But any hope I once had that I could talk with my patients in some detail, with personalized, one-on-one specificity, about the importance of eating certain foods and not eating certain other foods, and other ways to help themselves – forget it.

Prescribe, prescribe, prescribe.

Because primary care was now more or less built for it. As a primary care doctor, I had ten to fifteen minutes, max, with each patient, and virtually all of them came in with more than one problem. How can we adequately address all or even a couple of the crucial lifestyle issues in that sliver of time? So you give them prescriptions and get them on their way.

It would be one thing if this medication-first strategy usually worked. It doesn't. It often fails miserably. Meds band-aid the problem, not fix it. The next time the patient appears, he or she needs even more meds. So many of my patients continued to get worse. It was utterly depressing.

I wanted to be a doctor who, where possible, could *de*-prescribe medication for her patients. But that could happen only if I had time to talk and work with them in a meaningful way, and I didn't see how that was ever going to happen.

Day after day I came home to Brad, complaining. "I don't think I can make it to retirement this way," I told him. True, for years I had looked for a situation where I could be a doctor and also have a home life, and I had finally found it. In that way, primary care suited me.

But I was unfulfilled at work. I could feel myself getting more feisty and angry at a broken system.

~

Doctors want to make their patients happy. Doctors want their patients to like them.

As crazy as it sounds, those urges can cause a problem.

It was around this time that "Picker scores" were introduced nationally. After their office visits, patients were mailed a survey called the Picker Patient Experience Questionnaire to rate their doctors. The numbers tallied from the questionnaire – the Picker scores – could in turn affect a doctor's financial compensation, because pay was partly tied to them.

A bad score wasn't what rankled me; personally, I received good scores. No, what bothered me – infuriated me – was the incentive structure embedded in such a system. So many patients came to the offices of their primary care doctors wanting unwarranted antibiotics or pain medication, which often increased risk and obscured the bigger problem. But the doctor, knowing what the patient wanted, knowing it would make the patient happy to walk out of the office with a prescription, knowing the patient was more likely to rate the doctor higher because the patient got what he or she had come for, never mind the medical wisdom of it . . . I mean, how screwed up is that?

Our nation's tragic opioid crisis is in large part the direct result of patients wanting pain relief via medication, and doctors capitulating to that desire without time to consider the appropriateness or alternatives.

I grew more incensed about Picker scores when a paper published in a medical journal, *Archives of Internal Medicine*, reached the conclusion that patients who like their doctors are more likely to die.

Patients who like their doctors are more likely to die.

Let that sink in.

~

Enough was enough.

Once adorable Luna, our third, arrived and I returned from another eight-week maternity leave, I felt ready finally to tackle some of the work issues that had bothered me so much. Top of the list: medicine overprescription.

Because it wasn't just my colleagues at IUH who did it; it was true of the American healthcare system, generally. I called a contact at the IUH Pharmacy Department to see if, together, we could develop a protocol for advising physicians on appropriate antibiotic prescribing. One small step.

We had no template to work from, at least not one designed for a community like ours. Such protocols *had* been published in various medical journals – but that right there was the problem: no one paid attention to them. That's how we had gotten into this mess – no authoritative guidance. Essentially, overprescribing became the standard of care even though officially it wasn't. Standard of care means the commonly accepted treatment for a given condition. A better term here might be "dogma." It became dogma, and dogma is hard to break. Boy, would I learn that lesson hard in the upcoming years.

I wanted to create the new protocol in the right way, which meant doing it right for more than our small community, since the problem of abusing medication was much bigger than that. Why not engage others who could benefit? I contacted a friend who was a doctor at Franciscan Health, one of the three major healthcare organizations in Tippecanoe County, where we lived. I contacted another doctor from Unity Healthcare who was also the county health commissioner. These were our competitors for patients and business, essentially, but this wasn't about competition. (There is *so* much competition in health care, but in this particular case, thankfully, we were all able to transcend that.) Since I was talking to each of them, doctor to doctor, rather than organizational bureaucrat to organizational bureaucrat, it was easy to get them to agree to join the project.

I contacted local media outlets because none of this effort would amount to anything if people didn't know it existed, like those virtually invisible protocols published in medical journals. We held a press conference and explained what we were doing and why. Maybe more pivotal, all the doctors gathered there, from some of the major healthcare organizations in the county, vowed to bring the protocol back to all the physicians they worked with and get them to understand that these were the guidelines to follow. That would be huge. Sometimes, all a doctor needs is "cover." They could now turn down patient requests for unneeded medicine by saying, with a shrug, "Sorry, those are the rules'" or "My hands are tied," thus buying them time to gain a deeper understanding of the possible root of the problem. That, we felt, could have a profound effect on the numbers, and on how patients and doctors felt about medication. Doctors would worry less about getting crappy Picker scores from patients annoyed with them for depriving their immediate "fix," one that might be unhelpful and possibly even destructive.

I could tell the protocol was having an almost immediate effect because of a significant decrease in the volume of call requests. And I received lots of thank-you's from providers.

The whole experience was an eye-opening lesson in activism. Identify a real problem that most people know needs to change, yet one that nobody is doing anything to change because, well, status quo. Recruit stakeholders who agree with your position – for the same or different reasons – thus getting closer to Yes than No. For me, it was a triumph of what was possible if you're sufficiently angry and willing to try a new approach. That anger thing again.

I wished we had had the money to track metrics for the new protocol, so we knew with greater precision how well it was doing, and what we could do to improve it further. Unfortunately, the lack of resources for this kind of crucial follow-up hampers lots of great ideas from being even greater.

A few weeks after the protocol was put in place, one of the outpatient managers at IUH called. She was about to ask the question that launched the next chapter of my life.

"Sarah, we want to open a new obesity program here at IU," she said. "Would you be interested in heading it?"

~   ~   ~

PART 2

CHANGE THE WORLD

A wise man changes his mind, a fool never will.

- Proverb

Chapter 5

Rock My World

Yes, I would like to head up an obesity program. Very much so.

After seven years in primary care, I was burned out. Like so many people in health care, though, I also felt genuine concern for the problem of obesity – more accurately, the *epidemic* of obesity – and the many issues it touched on. It doesn't matter if you're a surgeon, a cardiologist, a primary care doctor, a dermatologist – so many patients walk into doctors' offices presenting a similar picture: overweight or obese and suffering from other chronic conditions, such as cholesterol abnormalities, kidney disease, hypertension, diabetes. In the previous couple of years I had said to anyone who would listen that we needed an obesity clinic on our IUH Arnett campus, because non-specialists had no time to deal with the real issues plaguing those with obesity. Primary care physicians had no meaningful chance to speak with these individuals at some compassionate length about necessary lifestyle changes. If doctors had more time, these issues could be addressed, with more positive results. I was sure of it.

IUH understood the need, too, and I give them credit for recognizing it. I never knew what made them decide to start the obesity program right then. Was it the success of the prescription protocol we had just rolled out? It didn't matter. The opportunity delighted me. I was ready for a change from the medicine I was practicing, and running an obesity clinic was at the top of the list. My hope was that we could treat obesity not just through medication but by getting at one of its deepest roots: nutrition.

Maybe it sounds odd to say that because, well, does it even need to be said? Treat obesity by tackling nutrition? Of *course* that's the key way to do it!

Unfortunately, even shockingly, that's not how obesity has been addressed, and to this day continues not to be addressed, by so many people who ought to know that fundamental fact. I can't tell you how many lectures, presentations, and discussions about obesity I've attended, where nutrition is lucky to get mentioned at all.

The focus, as always, is on prescription medication. And status quo thinking.

~

IUH was already running a conventional obesity program in Indianapolis, the only such program in the state at the time. It mostly featured a low-fat, low-calorie diet, or low-fat, low-cal meal replacements – shakes, protein bars, snacks, that sort of thing. I felt some pressure at least to start with something similar when our program opened.

I drove to Indy to meet the woman running the program, hoping for some guidance. She showed no interest in helping. I have no idea why. Our program would have to be created from scratch, based on what I would learn. Everything was on the table. The science, facts, evidence-based results – all this would rule the day – whatever they showed. The prospect terrified me for approximately forty-five seconds. Then I returned to my excitement about this huge opportunity.

What would our program encourage or discourage? What did other programs around the country do? What kind of success were they having? How did they measure success? What was the science behind it? Who were the best, smartest, most credible voices out there for new protocols? Would politics and bias be troublesome issues? Did self-interest on the part of organizations or individuals ever interfere with the most important idea out there – the patient's best interest? Had anyone solved the "unsolvable" health issue that is obesity?

What a gift this opportunity was. Practically no one gets a chance to do this, in the midst of a medical career: pause, read and study, consider, strategize. Doctors rarely get the chance. (*People* rarely get the chance.) I wanted to dive into the latest research, to understand the key issues at their root.

For the year ahead, IUH lightened my patient workload and paid for my courses and certifications so that I would have time to study and gain the credibility and authority needed to head a program under the auspices of a major medical institution. I had a year to spend with my nose in the literature.

I was already board-certified in internal medicine but now I prepped for my obesity boards, which meant lots of continuing medical education in obesity care, much of it in person, including attending conferences.

During the year, two of the many conferences I attended were run by the Obesity Medicine Association, which featured board review (think: preparing for the test) and numerous informative lectures, including by Dr. Steve Phinney and Dr. Jeff Volek, experts in and advocates for a low-carbohydrate diet. *Not low-fat but low-carb.*[2]

After hearing their first talk, I thought, *You know, that kind of makes sense.*

After hearing their second talk, I thought, *My god, that makes SO much sense.*

I asked one of the other conference attendees the best way to find out more about low-carb. "Is there a book I can read?" I asked.

"Jeff and Steve *wrote* the book," my colleague said, a reply as metaphorical as it was literal. "If you want to understand better, read the book."

I tracked down *The Art and Science of Low Carbohydrate Living* by Volek and Phinney, and read it that night. It was aimed at physicians.

It rocked my world.

I re-read the book.

I could call the lectures or the book my "Aha!" moment. But those few days at the conference were really my "Aha!" weekend, at the start of an "Aha!" year.

It was more than a shock to my system. Yes, what I heard and read made sense, but first I had to jettison what I had long believed. And what I believed

---

[2] The primary components of nutrition are the macronutrients — carbohydrates, fats, and proteins. They provide the calories needed for energy plus materials needed for growth and repair. See the Glossary for details about carbohydrates.

was what so much of the medical establishment and general public had long believed: that low-fat and low-calorie were the way to go.

When you're confronted with an idea that seems right – scientifically, logically sound – and yet it also goes against what you have believed for so long, a belief whose science you may simply have presumed because, well, everyone taught you that it was true . . . when you come to such a fork in the road, your belief system finds itself in crisis. Your first inclination is to deny. To push back. To insist that what you have always believed to be true must still be, and that this new counter-idea must have obvious holes in it that you just don't see yet. There *has* to be some faulty, intellectual bias to the new idea that will reveal itself. Because, hey, the status quo is the status quo for a reason, right? If the status quo were wrong, perhaps spectacularly wrong, no way could it have just sat around this long, unchallenged by those in authority, unchecked by smart, caring, informed people, no way could it have just remained in place, harming countless people, profoundly, every day, for decades . . . right? How could that be?

Okay, fine, New Idea may work under certain very particular conditions but, but – well, it can't be right, generally. It can't! . . . can it?

It's tough to challenge yourself with any new idea. By doing so, you're opening up the possibility that you – and possibly many others, including people you respect – have been wrong, and wrong for a long time, with a potential trail of damage for having believed and espoused the wrong ideas and advice. If you're a doctor, maybe you yourself shared your fallacious ideas with patients, who took it as gospel and made life changes based on these fallacious ideas. I thought of my patients back when I was an exercise physiologist, such as my cardiac patient Ken, and how the only nutritional advice I knew then was

low calorie = good
low fat = good

It's a strange feeling to realize you've been wrong about something so fundamental to your life. It doesn't feel good. It's embarrassing. There's a lot of guilt.

My transformation was gradual but undeniable.

Holy cow, I've been wrong for a really long time.

More self-questioning.

And then I got – naturally – angry.

I wondered: *How could people – doctors, researchers, scientists! – say things unsupported by evidence?*

That's about where I was, from late 2011 through late 2012. When I wasn't seeing patients in a more limited capacity (I was down to three days a week instead of five), I was reading everything I could on the subjects of diet, nutrition, obesity, diabetes, insulin resistance,[3] and much more. I was forced to think more deeply about the physiology behind nutrition. I read and studied, giving the new idea – that nutrition-influenced health outcomes are at least as much about carbohydrate

---

[3] Insulin is a hormone your pancreas releases to enable cells in your body to absorb blood sugar (glucose) to be used for energy. For many people the cells do not operate normally and they resist using the insulin; so we say they are insulin resistant. Insulin resistance varies among individuals and is a primary factor in obesity and diabetes. See the Glossary for further details.

intake as fat intake or calorie intake – an equal shot at being right. I identified more presumptions I had been toting around for years, like exercising to lose weight or counting calories or the role of LDL cholesterol, turning these ideas over to see if they, too, had possibly rested on a faulty premise and shaky evidence.

That's how I came to understand that a low-fat diet – with its high carbohydrate corollary – makes zero physiological sense for anyone with insulin resistance. That includes, I now knew, most people with obesity, everyone with type 2 diabetes, and many people without diabetes as well.

Zero sense. As in, none.

And it is estimated that about a third of American adults are insulin resistant.

Yet I was still not a full convert to low carb. For all my willingness to look in the mirror, I still didn't know enough. I did literature searches, read every research study I could find on the topic, actively sought out more and more information. I read deeply on the subject of carbohydrate restriction. Although I was starting to embrace ideas touted by the "low-carb community," I knew it was important to maintain objectivity: After all, I'd just had my world rocked by the realization that the science I thought was valid, wasn't, so I needed to be as well-read as possible in other related areas, such as lipids (think cholesterol and fats). I planned to get board-certified in lipidology, too, to strengthen my understanding of the physiology of human nutrition. I needed to understand better how our bodies use nutrients from food and how we produce energy and store fat. All this would give me needed credibility for when I inevitably went up against old-school, status quo forces who resisted changing their minds regardless of the evidence growing before their eyes. It was a replay of the reason I got into medicine.

Remember Dr. Conklin, the pompous ass who had dismissed me and others like me because he felt that only doctors knew what was really going on? And whose demeaning, know-it-all attitude inspired me then and there to show him and others like him where they were wrong? Well, that time had come. Now, two decades later, I would make sure that I was at least as informed as – ideally, more informed than – those with whom I disagreed. I wasn't trying to be the smartest one in the room. This was simply a sensible, science-backed way to approach issues. And since I wanted to win over as many people as possible, using science and facts was the best way to do it. If what I subsequently learned in lipidology led me to other conclusions? So be it.

Before my thinking morphed, I had thought that our obesity clinic would start off featuring a low-fat, calorie-restricted diet. Now? *No way*. Based on the work by Phinney and Volek that became my diet bible; that of science journalists Gary Taubes and Nina Teicholz; Dr. Eric Westman, director of the Duke Keto Medicine Clinic, and others, it was becoming clear that the only conclusion you could make about the low-fat diet was that it was a provably abject failure.

On the other hand, there was real evidence supporting the benefits of a low-carb diet despite the lengths to which supporters of the status quo would go to resist it. My investigation into the literature found that the simple approach of decreasing carbohydrates and increasing fat in the diet helps people lose weight *without counting calories, without even instructing them to eat less*. And it positively impacts other aspects of metabolic health,[4] such as lowering cardiovascular risk and improving diabetes.

I envisioned a program where patients could largely keep their eating pattern preferences after they were educated about substitutions. If you're vegetarian or vegan? Yep, you could keep to either diet while also lowering your carbs, though vegans would need to be attentive to their consumption of essential nutrients. If you wanted to keep to cultural eating patterns – Mexican, Korean, Indian, Italian, you name it? That was also possible, with some low-carb education.

I decided to try the low-carb diet myself.

For years Brad had been saying about himself, "I can't eat carbs." They made him feel listless, he said, as well as (my favorite) "puffy." For years I'd been poking fun at him. "You're being ridiculous," I told him.

Now that I was reading the science on it, I changed my tune. Brad had been right the whole time (and, much to his delight, I told him so)! What he felt was absolutely real, though not everyone was affected by carbs the way he was – he had a family history of insulin resistance while I did not. I had what I thought was a pretty healthy diet to start. Brad and I had always eaten lots of veggies, a good amount of protein, and fruit. Our diet was, naturally, low-fat – lean meats, low-fat dairy, not much butter or bacon, and such. I quickly realized that this new low-carb regimen did not have to

---

[4] Metabolism refers to the breakdown of food and its conversion to energy for the body. It is a major factor in obesity and diabetes and other chronic diseases. You will be seeing the terms metabolism, metabolic health, metabolic disease, and metabolic syndrome throughout this book. See the Glossary for details.

be a burden. Let me type those words again: this new eating regimen did not have to be a burden. It was not about starvation because *I did not have to restrict calories*. I didn't have to try and eat less. I could eat as much as I wanted by just avoiding carbohydrate-rich foods.

And it tasted good because I had a substantial amount of fat in my diet, and fat is a flavor carrier. The smells and texture of fatty foods add to their attraction.[5] Plus, I flavored my food with one or more of the many seasonings in our herb cabinet. Having your own herb garden is not mandatory for eating flavorful healthy food, though Brad and I had had such a garden since our first house.

The low-carb diet fit in with my normal living because I wasn't thinking about it all the time.

I responded well enough that I took the next step, and Brad joined me: a full-on ketogenic diet – a very low-carb diet decidedly high in fats, with enough protein too. With a well-formulated ketogenic, or "keto," diet, where your daily carbohydrate intake is under 50 grams, fat from both ingested and stored fat is converted into ketone "bodies," which become a major energy source, rather than blood sugar, the predominant energy source from a high-carb diet. It may come as a surprise but you can run your body mostly on carbs (blood sugar) . . . or you can run it

---

[5] Our preference for and consumption of fats may be an evolutionary phenomenon, responsible for the development of the human brain: Montmayeur JP, le Coutre J, editors. *Fat Detection: Taste, Texture, and Post Ingestive Effects.* Chapter 1: Leonard WR, Snodgrass JJ, Robertson ML. *Evolutionary Perspectives on Fat Ingestion and Metabolism in Humans.* ncbi.nlm.nih.gov/books/NBK53561/

mostly on fats (ketones)._[6]

Later, after I launched the obesity clinic and people found out that I, at a low-normal weight, was following a ketogenic diet, they always asked me why. My answer was always the same.

1. I do it for my patients, to understand more of what they're experiencing on the road to getting healthier. You can't teach it as well if you don't live it.
2. I do it because it's part of my plan to stay fit. Low carb doesn't just benefit those who are overweight or diabetic; slim and otherwise healthy people can be pre- or diabetic and it is a good way to eat to maintain good metabolic health
3. I do it as a model for my children. If they don't overdo carbs – especially sugar – while growing up, they will be much more likely to enter adulthood without the need for severe dietary restrictions on carbohydrates for people who have developed insulin resistance and then obesity or diabetes._[7]

Though I was always slender, I still lost weight on the low-carb and ketogenic diets.

I gained considerable muscle mass (IUH bought a body composition analyzer for the clinic). I could see

---

[6] See the Glossary for details about the ketogenic diet and ketones.

[7] Yes, they still have (some) Halloween candy and birthday cakes, but over all the kids don't consume nearly as many carbs as the American norm. And they aren't all that attracted to candy and sugary things. A good start for preventing metabolic disease.

the improvement myself.

Maybe most important: I passed my obesity boards.

~

Want to hear some shocking things I learned from my immersion in the science behind nutrition, health, weight, and obesity?

Studies show that full-fat dairy is not associated with obesity in children any more than low-fat dairy and some studies even show that full-fat dairy consumption is *less* likely to lead to childhood obesity.

Wait . . . what?

Crazy, right? How can that be?

Because the low-fat diet is a sham.

Yogurt is the classic example.

There is nothing redeeming about low-fat yogurt. Please let that sink in. The fat naturally in yogurt is removed. With less fat, the flavor needs to be made more palatable and is replaced with carbs, including a ridiculous amount of sugar in flavored yogurt. More carbs and less fat means people get hungry quicker. A health-conscious, weight-conscious individual is far better served by buying whole-fat yogurt, adding (for example) a tablespoon of real peanut butter (no sugar or other additives except perhaps salt), and mixing together those two whole foods. It tastes good. It has no added sugar. And because it has plenty of fat, you feel full afterward. A few berries, vanilla extract, dark chocolate or cocoa, or unsweetened coconut, are also fine, flavorful additions. Monk fruit or other sweetener can also be added.

It was a challenge to get patients to accept eating

fat, to get over the ingrained fat phobia. Even in our household the low-fat regimen was hard to break. It took six months to get the kids off fat-free milk and onto whole milk. We brought butter back into the home. You can imagine how much better things tasted. And bacon!

I know, I know: What about the restriction on *saturated* fat? For decades, many prominent health organizations have insisted that we need to restrict saturated fat. Why? Well, they say, saturated fats lead to higher cholesterol, especially LDL cholesterol,[8] and that leads to increased cardiovascular risk (think heart attacks). And of course eating fat means you'll gain weight, right? But the recommendation on saturated fat wasn't based on evidence. It wasn't when the original recommendation was issued and it isn't now.

No evidence.

Let *that* sink in.

Do you know where the recommended ceilings on saturated fat came from?

Nowhere. They were made up. Totally arbitrary. The evidence to support a restriction on saturated fat is not there, and never was. It's a scam. (Too harsh? Just wait until you hear its origin story.)

Yet the federal government's Dietary Guidelines for Americans (DGA) still recommends a diet low in fat, especially low in saturated fat – and, as a result, high in carbohydrates. The DGA (which I'll call the Guidelines) were born in 1977 when the Senate Select Committee on Nutrition and Human Needs issued a report titled "Dietary Goals for the United States," with

---

[8] LDL is often referred to as the "bad" cholesterol. HDL is the "good" cholesterol. They are sometimes given as LDL-C and HDL-C. See the Glossary for details.

recommendations that, boiled down, advised this: eat less; eat less fat, especially saturated; eat more complex carbohydrates and "natural" sugars (such as fruit juice! no!), with a limit on added sugar of 10% (that's a lot!) of your daily calories. Oh, and exercise more.

In 1980, the US Department of Health and Human Services (HHS) and the US Department of Agriculture (USDA) took over the recommendations and began to issue the Guidelines. The Guidelines are updated every five years, providing "advice on what to eat and drink to meet nutrient needs, promote health, and prevent disease." Although the HHS description states that "[e]ach edition of the Dietary Guidelines reflects the current body of nutrition science," the research and studies on low-carbohydrate versus low-fat have been ignored.

The 2020-2025 Guidelines do not recommend a "low-fat diet," but in their list of recommended foods, they include fat-free or low-fat milk, yogurt, and cheese, and lean meats. Odd. Obviously components of a low-fat diet. They specifically warn about saturated fat, which, they say, should be less than 10% of calories.

Why would this be? Well, many of the people on the Dietary Guidelines Committee are nutrition scientists – usually, mainstream nutrition scientists. Status quo nutrition scientists. For the most recent update, one committee member had done a trial on low-carbohydrate nutrition, but she seemed to have little impact on the final recommendations; perhaps (to be fair) she influenced the rest of them from making recommendations which were even more disappointing.

In the end, the key message that the Guidelines perpetuated: Fat is bad! You don't want to be fat, so don't eat fat! Fat has twice the calories per gram, so it must be dangerous!

All wrong!

(Could the association between consuming fat and being fat have all been avoided if fat – dietary fat – merely had a different name? I have often wondered that.)

Because of the arbitrary, evidence-free, recommended caps on saturated fat, you cannot meet nutrient sufficiency (such as various amino acids, fatty acids, vitamins, and minerals that have to be consumed because the body does not produce them, or not enough of them), not even close, by following the Guidelines, unless you also follow its other key recommendations: eat highly processed and refined grains. Because most foods containing saturated fat happen to be very nutrient-dense, there would be no need to consume these grains on a high-fat diet.

Let's talk about those refined grains. Note first that at least a third of adult Americans are insulin resistant. Being insulin resistant means your body cannot handle all the blood sugar that is produced when it breaks down the carbohydrates you have consumed; so blood sugar (glucose) rises beyond normal levels after eating and/or does not come back down to normal levels.[9] The Guidelines recommend five to six servings of refined grains, which is just about the *worst* food to eat if you're insulin resistant. So why do people eat it? Maybe more to the point, why is this recommended? Because those grains are *fortified* – vitamins are added – thus fulfilling some of an individual's daily nutrient

---

[9] High blood sugar is the biomarker for diabetes. See the Glossary for details about diabetes.

needs. Amazingly, even if you were to consume the amount of refined and processed grains that the Guidelines recommend, you would *still* be short on necessary nutrients.

I need to repeat this because it's so big and scary: to get you close to being nutrient-sufficient, our government recommends that you eat grains that are refined and processed, *which worsens a condition you may well have.*

We should be suspicious of any dietary guidelines where you can't meet your needs with whole foods alone. Whole foods are not refined or processed (or only minimally) and have no added ingredients, especially no artificial ingredients. Eggs, fresh produce, nuts, fresh fish and meat, for example, are whole foods. Eating these kinds of whole foods is the way people ate for most of human existence, and as far as we know *they did not die of nutrition-related diseases* (other than starvation: lack of food overall). Today, we *do* die because of our nutrition. Rampantly. There are many examples of the following truth, including those published in peer-reviewed medical literature: a carbohydrate-restricted, whole-food diet can easily meet nutrient sufficiency, so long as you ignore the ridiculous, fictional cap on saturated fat.

~

Studying the world of nutrition exposed me to other examples of how scientific evidence was ignored when it did not align with the status quo. Take a huge clinical trial called the Women's Health Initiative. Those for whom that phrase registers might say, "Oh, right! The study that showed most women shouldn't be on Hormone Replacement Therapy (HRT) because it can do more harm than good." And they would be right. That was a good recommendation. Generally, women shouldn't be on HRT.[10] That's the takeaway that made for big headlines.

Yet that was not the only objective of the study. Guess what else was? Showing a relationship between dietary fat and heart disease (also between dietary fat and breast and colon cancers). The National Institutes of Health (NIH) invested hundreds of millions of dollars to fund a study that would show how a low-fat diet decreases the risk of heart disease and some cancers.[11]

Except that the study did no such thing. No correlation was found between dietary fat and heart disease, breast cancer, or colon cancer.[12] Even though

---

[10] Editor's note: Despite the headlines about HRT, estrogen or estrogen/progesterone therapy is appropriate for treating serious symptoms for some women transitioning to menopause. The WHI study found that these hormone treatments should *not* be used as a preventative for chronic diseases including cardiovascular disease and invasive breast cancer, among others. They are ineffective and have their own risks. See: Thomson C, Anderson G. For the Women's Health Initiative Steering Committee. *News from the WHI Study: WHI Response to NYT article "Women have been misled about menopause."* 2/15/2023.
www.whi.org/md/news/nyt-response

[11] NIH, $625m, "the largest single research study to be funded by NIH." The funding was split among several components of the study, not just the diet modification arm. Institute of Medicine (US) Committee to Review the NIH Women's Health Initiative; Thaul S, Hotra D, editors. "An Assessment of the NIH Women's Health Initiative." 1993.
ncbi.nlm.nih.gov/books/NBK236506/

[12] The study was conducted on postmenopausal women ages 50 to 79. Howard BV, Van Horn L, Hsia J, Manson JE, et al. "Low-fat dietary pattern and risk of cardiovascular disease: the Women's Health

the study was published, *that* part barely made the news. What *was* publicized? The finding about HRT, an admittedly important one.

But an important part of the study went bust. And for a long time, no one bothered to say anything.

~ ~ ~

Initiative Randomized Controlled Dietary Modification Trial." *JAMA* 2006 Feb 8;295(6):655-66.
pubmed.ncbi.nlm.nih.gov/16467234/
The study also did not find any correlation between the low-fat diet and either breast or colon cancer. Prentice RL, Caan B, Chlebowski RT, Patterson R, Kuller LH, et al. "Low-fat dietary pattern and risk of invasive breast cancer: the Women's Health Initiative Randomized Controlled Dietary Modification Trial." *JAMA*. 2006 Feb 8;295(6):629-42.
pubmed.ncbi.nlm.nih.gov/16467232/

Chapter 6

Team Spirit, Patient Success

In the fall of 2012, we launched the obesity program –
officially, the IU Health Arnett Medically Supervised
Weight Loss Clinic (now the IU Health Arnett
Physicians Medical Weight Loss). That fall was a time
of lots of meetings and planning. Our team formed
quickly. I was able to hire Joni, my former medical
assistant extraordinaire, and we were thrilled to be
working together again. Patti McKee was a medical
assistant in the primary care clinic and we were lucky to
bring her on our team. Monica Keyes, a nurse
practitioner, started working for the clinic one day a
week, but showed such interest in obesity issues and
was so good at what she did that we soon hired her full
time. Danielle Wharff, an RN, joined us soon after and
was instrumental in dealing with educational materials
and patient rewards. Zach Roberts, a medical assistant,
came on board a little after that and among other things
assisted with the computer side of things. The whole
team was amazing, each as enthusiastic about what
could be accomplished as I was.

I had learned enough in the previous year that I
was confident we ought to start as a carbohydrate-
restricted program. Monica and I visited Eric
Westman's Duke Keto Medicine Clinic in North
Carolina to observe a very low-carb obesity clinic in

action. It was there that we hit on the idea of group sessions that were to become such an important motivating force in our own clinic. Eric also rewarded his "50-pound losers" with special recognition – he played the loser's favorite song on the piano. That's what I call a winner. Unfortunately, I'm a bit (okay, very) short-changed when it comes to things musical. So we were more traditional – awarding gifts of water bottles and lunch bags – but our patients were enthusiastic.

We were given space in the primary care clinic. We designated our most important physical area "the education room," where we all would provide information and answer questions for patients in groups. Members of the staff were not just staff, they were educators.

I told my team that I didn't just want to push the ideas that I had learned over the past year. I wanted to hear what they had to say, what they had learned, what they might want to add. When someone made a suggestion, I acknowledged it; even if the idea was something that didn't work, or that we ultimately didn't implement, we were a team, not a hierarchy. I had seen how ideas communicated forcefully could overwhelm the truth of those ideas. That wasn't going to be us.

Before our "soft open" in early 2013, I started attending every medical department meeting in the IUH Arnett system, across almost every medical specialty, and gave a 15-minute slide presentation explaining what we planned on doing at the clinic and why it made scientific sense. This was necessary because, at the time, the benefit of the low-carb diet was still a relatively new "theory," at least for our geographic area.

I needed to get ahead of the confusion that would surely ensue when patients returned to their primary care providers and announced, "Dr. Hallberg told me to eat lots of fat!" The presentations extended into the full opening of the clinic later in 2013.

I hoped these presentations would help all the physicians, nurses, and medical staff see what I saw. I told them, "I know some of your patients who are in our weight-loss clinic told you that I encouraged them to eat more fat, and you think I'm crazy." It always got a modest laugh. "Well, I'm not, and here's why." At the end of my presentation, I transferred some of the burden to them. "Not only is there evidence for the low-carb diet, but it's on all of us to make that fact known to all patients being treated at IUH, for any type of metabolic disease.[13] They should understand it's an option."

Many of my lectures started with a slide outlining the three clinically proven ways to treat obese patients:

Option 1: bariatric surgery

Option 2: extreme low-calorie diet (we're talking 700-900 calories a day)

Option 3: low-carbohydrate diet

Once the audience had taken in the information, I would ask, "Which option is supported by the most evidence?"

The answer: bariatric surgery.

---

[13] Metabolic disease is a broad designation for a metabolism-related condition that is the basis of many chronic diseases. See the Glossary for details about Metabolic Disease, Metabolic Syndrome and Metabolism.

Many patients choose this option, while many others are frightened by the idea of undergoing surgery. It's also very expensive, but cost has really come down now that a gastric sleeve has become the most frequently performed surgery. There may be postoperative complications, though far fewer than in the past. The biggest problem with bariatric surgery? It is not changing eating patterns. It is not teaching people that their metabolic disease can be treated with food and that this treatment can bring meaningful improvement and even disease reversal. In the end, bariatric surgery is not the answer for the majority of obese individuals. But it must be acknowledged that it can work, and that there are people for whom it is the right option. It's certainly not my wish to see this option disappear.

What about the other two options?

An extreme calorie-restricted diet succeeds for a while – until it doesn't. It's well-documented that people can't continue it for very long; severely low caloric intake is unsustainable. You can experience short-term weight loss with an extreme low-calorie diet, but the only way to sustain the weight loss is to stay low-calorie forever – in effect, to always be hungry – or switch to a carbohydrate-restricted diet (option #3). And if *that's* the case, then why not follow the much easier route of a low-carb diet from the outset?

As much as I tried to educate patients and medical professionals about what I'd been learning, there were so many very smart, obvious questions that my staff and I fielded constantly.

Isn't cholesterol bad for your heart?
How can I possibly stick with this diet?
Isn't this a fad diet?

Isn't fruit important?

What will my cardiologist say?

How can I lose weight if I'm not counting calories?

To their credit, the doctors around me at IUH got it. They were smart; they appreciated evidence; most of them just hadn't had time in their busy lives to pause and think about the science of carbs and fat before I got in their faces. Once I put it out there, they saw it made sense, and was scientifically supported.

Patients started coming to the clinic. Each of them took part in a group meeting in the education room, where I gave a 45-minute lecture, with slides, explaining the physiology behind the low-carb philosophy. I made sure always to say, "I won't tell you what to eat. I want to help you understand why certain choices are better than others." I talked about nutrition and insulin physiology. It was a pretty in-depth lecture. I felt it was important for patients to understand the science.

In the early moments of my presentations to patients, I often saw confusion or skepticism in their eyes and expressions. As I delved deeper, I could see the light go on. Many of them would come up to me afterward and say some version of, "Wow, that makes sense." It reminded me of me, when I first heard Steve Phinney and Jeff Volek lecturing. The patients I addressed were deeply grateful that a doctor was pausing to explain something vital to their long-term well-being. They were grateful that the team and I listened and addressed their questions. They were grateful that we were giving them more than ninety seconds and a scribbled script. And I was so grateful to

71

be part of all this. This was a huge step for patients, making a very difficult lifestyle change; if it was easy, everyone would do it. They were allowing me to walk this journey with them. It was a privilege that I was honored, at times almost overwhelmed, to be given.

Maybe more than anything, what struck me was how everyone who came to these meetings – it didn't matter their education level, age, income; I mean *everyone* – got it. Which validated a thought I had long carried around, and that my years in medicine had only confirmed:

Doctors can be narcissists.

So many doctors have this notion that boils down to, "Oh, forget going into detail with that poor, stupid patient because she/he can't understand." That's what they often say, in different ways, when patients aren't around, and not infrequently when they are.

They won't get it.

Dumb it down.

Just tell them what they absolutely need to know. They don't need to know the rest.

Here I was, explaining advanced physiology to women and men brave enough to come to our clinic, and *every single person there got it*. You can explain this science to anyone.

It was yet another "Aha!" moment. It revealed another fundamental truth that medicine had gotten wrong for so long. We disrespect patients and undersell their intellectual capabilities. It's insulting, it's ridiculous, it's counterproductive, *it's based on a false understanding of people.*

During those early days of the clinic, it was this realization that motivated me, more even than the notion that we had gotten the dietary recommendations wrong for so long. It was the fact that we had minimized patients' ability to:

(a) learn and understand basic information, and

(b) stick with a program if they were given good clear advice, with supportive follow-up and an understanding of why making changes made sense.

In fairness, doctors usually don't have the time or the educational materials that we had to explain the patient's condition in depth. (But still.)

That was the moment I felt myself transforming, if subtly, from being a physician to a patient advocate. *All* physicians should be patient advocates. Not all of us are.

~   ~   ~

Chapter 7

It's Not the Patient's Fault

A morbidly obese man in his 20s came to my office. He showed me a photograph of his parents and siblings: each one thin, not a hint of weight issues. He had struggled professionally, struggling to find himself. He was single. Obviously his obesity affected his physical health but it affected everything else as well. Where did he believe he "fit" in his family? Our conversation was partly about his feeling like a black sheep. About his need to feel an identity that was not first and foremost about being "the fat one," the outlier.

But how would he? His early identity had shaped every aspect of his life. (To be fair, our early identity does that for all of us, weight issues or not.) How did that impression of himself – imposed from the outside, then cemented internally – impede his success at work? We had to do more than help him "just" with dietary changes; he needed to appreciate himself and find a path forward.

It is not unusual in obesity medicine to deal with more than diet. I had worked with enough obese, often extremely obese, patients to feel that I understood the psychological, emotional, and practical issues they frequently faced. We often had one-on-one conversations as a way to get patients to talk it out. Sometimes I was able to help them recognize what was going on and how to get to a better place. At times I referred them to a mental health counselor. We took our patients' mental health as seriously as the physical.

How difficult and horrible is it for an individual who struggles with obesity to grow up and live in a family of rail-thin people, raised under the same roof, eating more or less the same foods? How much shame and internal toil does that person feel? Lots of people around him will say it's got to be his fault; after all, look how everyone else is able to control themselves! What torture.

Clearly there *was* something different about this young man. When we blame the one suffering (we do this with lots of conditions, but obesity is just about the worst), we miss the real culprit: biology. People with weight issues or obesity are in a constant battle with their bodies. Their bodies essentially think they are always in a state of starvation due (most often) to insulin resistance. For people with insulin resistance, after consuming carbohydrates, which break down into blood sugar, their bodies produce more and more insulin. Insulin is a fat storage hormone and it also drives hunger.[14]

This "perceived" starvation drives hunger and cravings. I mean, if you're starving, you should eat, right? If that's not bad enough, what the body is craving makes things worse. People who are high-carbohydrate consumers don't crave a steak or a salad drenched in fatty dressing; they want simple carbohydrates. Simple

---

[14] When insulin is resisted and cells do not absorb all the blood sugar produced by the breakdown of carbohydrates, the "excess" sugar is converted to fat by the liver and fat cells. That's why we say that insulin is a fat storage hormone.

carbohydrates are often referred to as "readily available," meaning they are a quick source of energy, the fuel for high-carbohydrate consumers. As more carbohydrates are consumed, blood sugar goes up and insulin goes up in response, making it easy for the body to store fat, especially for someone who is insulin resistant. I've had many people describe it as if they are almost separated from their body, as if they have absolutely no control over how much they are eating. This is NOT – I repeat NOT – about lack of willpower.

Obesity does not discriminate. Women and men both struggle with it. It hits all ethnic groups, though certain populations, particularly Latinos, Pacific Islanders, American Indians, and African Americans suffer more. The affluent and highly educated may have a lower risk profile, but that doesn't mean that many members of that cohort won't become overweight. Because some will. No demographic category is immune.

In our clinic, we had many men and women in the range of 300-400+ pounds coming to us for help. They had family members saying, basically, that it was their own fault – they just ate too much. Some patients had trouble getting in and out of the car for their doctor visits. Drivers and passersby looked at them as if they were clearly to blame for their predicament.

Unjustified, stigmatizing blame and fault are thrown around all the time. Dangerously. Unfairly. For example: evidence suggests that losing weight is harder for women, especially postmenopausal, and we're not sure why, a frustration for patients and medical providers alike.[15] It doesn't help that some doctors will hear a female patient claim that she has struggled mightily to lose weight since menopause, then downplay or discredit her contention, or even demean her, telling her she's crazy or misguided; that there's nothing about her new situation that prevents her from losing weight at the same rate as she did before. "Just don't eat so much!" is the simplistic recommendation.

But it's *clearly* more difficult! Just because we have yet to determine *why* doesn't make it less true, or their struggles less real. Maddeningly, this attitude on the part of doctors happens often. It's unhelpful and unkind. Because medicine doesn't yet understand something, it must be the patient's fault? That's not very scientific. The best advice I gave to the many women who told me these stories: find a different doctor.

Typically, when people "go on a diet," they reduce their calorie intake, probably cut down on fat, and maybe they exercise. They may succeed in losing weight, but they find it difficult to keep off. Why? During their dieting, the calorie restriction and exercise will decrease their metabolic rate, a natural reflex of the body to conserve calories. But the slower rate lasts even when they regain weight, which puts them in a *worse* situation than when they started. This was well demonstrated in a scientific follow-up study on a contestant on the TV show, *The Biggest Loser*. In that case, the contestant rapidly lost 239 pounds on a

---

[15] Why women have a harder time than men losing weight, or even if they really do, is an area of controversy. There are many possible explanations, including differences in muscle mass, where fat is stored (apple v. pear shape), the decrease in estrogen over time for women, different metabolic rates, and losing weight at different rates. In the meantime, let's not blame them.

restricted calorie diet and intense daily activity. Afterwards, like many of the other contestants who had quickly lost significant amounts of weight, he gradually regained much of the weight (100 pounds), partly because of his decreased metabolism, and partly because of a typical reduction in his diet habits of what he ate and how much he exercised. Now he can consume no more than 800 calories a day to keep from regaining still more. Another argument against "just eat less and exercise more."

This is why, in our clinic, I say, "'Diet' is a four-letter word. We're doing lifestyle change."

My morbidly obese young patient lost weight – a lot of weight. He is not thin, but he is now in control. Carbohydrate restriction helped him reverse the level of insulin resistance that was behind his weight problem. Less resistance means less insulin is produced, and because insulin is a fat storage hormone, less fat is stored. Some relief for him, at last.

~

Now and then a patient had a problem that required my taking him or her out of the group for a heart-to-heart. The problem rarely concerned a dietary recommendation. It was a crisis involving family or something equally major. I was able to do what I so rarely could in my previous life as primary care physician: sit with my patient, give counsel, provide support.

The most common problem I encountered involved patients taking care of aging or sick parents. The average age of our patients was 54 years and many of them were deeply involved in the care of one or two quite aged parents. There were also crises involving the health of a spouse or their children, job loss, or other major life change. When you're burdened by such a circumstance, it's harder than normal to work on changing yourself.

I wasn't a trained therapist but I knew this simple truth: when people are upset, they want to be heard, they want their feelings to be acknowledged. And what they often feel is shame.

If an overweight person is caring for a parent, for example, and that parent needs to go to the hospital, and the caretaker is presented with no particularly healthy food options because hospitals are notoriously terrible about the food they provide (seriously?!), and the hungry caretaker ends up eating something she wouldn't otherwise choose, she's not yet trained to tell herself, *I'm in the hospital with my mother, she's dying, it's an all-around crappy situation, and I ate a potato because that was all that was available, and it's okay because tomorrow I'll do better.*

No. Instead, she says something like, *I ate a potato and I'm a terrible, horrible human being.* In situations like this, part of our role was to get patients to talk it out, to acknowledge that they were suffering from shame, to which I would say, in essence, "Now look here . . . "

Here is a dramatic, but not unusual, example of what I mean: a patient I'll call Carol was walking through the mall, saw the reflection of a woman in a store window, and thought, "Oh wow! She's a good weight."

A surreal instant later, Carol realized it was her own reflection.

She found the nearest bench and began to sob. They weren't tears of happiness. Carol cried because she realized that the very first judgment she made about this "stranger" concerned weight. Her first thought was, *Oh, that person's not fat.* She was ashamed of judging people that way. She was ashamed for judging herself that way. She realized, in what should have been a triumphant moment, that every time in her life up to that one, when she looked in the mirror she never once thought of herself as not fat. "Fat" is such a pejorative word in our culture; individuals using it to describe themselves is part of the shame many feel.

I began regularly telling that story (with Carol's blessing) to others with weight struggles. For me, it was a perfect illustration of how profoundly hard it is to lose weight *and* lose the sense of yourself as a "fat" person. When you've seen yourself as overweight your whole life, losing weight is not the only thing you need to do. There are emotional and psychological issues to address and work through, as well. In our clinic, we tried to help our patients deal with those issues.

We sometimes also had to cope with the fact that families and friends might not be supportive of our patients' dietary changes. I remember one man who had knee problems because of his weight, even after replacement of both knees. He lost 40 pounds in our clinic but his wife kept undermining him with comments like, "Oh, he doesn't have to be that restrictive" or "He can have fries sometimes." After a while, he dropped out, regained the 40 pounds and then some, and went back to having trouble walking. This scenario reminded me of the undermining some of my college classmates had to put up with when family urged them to stop their schooling and "get a real job already."

Society can be cruel about weight issues. So can one's own family and loved ones. So can one's doctors and other healthcare professionals. Changing diet while living in a household of non-dieters can be incredibly difficult for the dieter. The others in the home might not want to make changes in their own diets, which can then make meals and trips to the kitchen a temptation and torture.

Obviously, lifestyle changes are multi-faceted. It's almost never just one thing. It's genetics. It's age. It's environment. It's time of life. But nutrition is so, so crucial, and for far too long it has been misunderstood, in large part because it's been badly, often deceptively, "explained."

And let's face it: carbs are everywhere. We live in a carb-centric world.

~   ~   ~

Chapter 8

Rock My World, Again

At the clinic, the patient was given the choice of a low-carb, whole foods diet free of processed food, or meal replacements. We included the meal replacements early on only because that's what they'd done before at IUH, and it was the prevailing wisdom at weight-loss clinics around the country, even as I believed by then that it was a scientifically unsound (read "worthless") regimen.

And soon enough, we eliminated that option. Because the evidence said so. I knew the results of well-managed clinical trials. Meal replacements did not work and do not work long-term for the vast majority, simple as that. People need to eat *real* food while they're losing weight. The rate of weight regain on a replacement meal plan is ridiculously high. People then blame themselves for a failure that is not theirs. They aren't learning to eat properly to control their health. There's a lot of money to be made from replacement meals – that's why they're still around – but their long-term health value is minimal. Meal replacements only postpone the inevitable; no one stays on them forever. Everyone in our office agreed with eliminating them. The medical assistants had as much input as I did. It was a collaborative environment.

Soon, we had almost more patients than we could handle. I was giving my explanatory presentation five times a week. The team and I took note of what seemed to work in our approach and what didn't, and we constantly made changes, big and small.

It wasn't long before I noticed a serious problem, one that struck at the heart of what I had so not liked about primary care: The more patients we had, the less one-on-one time each of them could get.

So we doubled down on group gatherings. While one-on-one time can be useful and often essential, group meetings allowed us so much more time in each other's presence. I really got to know everyone; they got to know me far better than if we'd had only very occasional one-on-ones. And the best thing about group meetings: the participants got to know each other. The support everyone felt was tremendous. Even the quieter people would eventually talk. It was better that we were doing it in groups.

Another recommendation that made us different: we discouraged patients who were not currently exercising from starting right away. To tell someone who weighs 350 pounds to go and exercise, when he or she hasn't done so in a very long time, is to invite great risk. And when patients hurt themselves, they're usually going to quit – not just quit exercise but quit other regimens that have the potential to improve their health. Of course, we wanted to encourage a positive health care environment, but abiding by the physician's credo to "First do no harm," we also needed to lower the risk of a negative environment. Pushing non-exercisers suddenly to exercise, thus inviting the not-insignificant risk of injury, felt almost punitive. Instead, we told the more obese patients, "You can exercise sometime in the future – not now." I thought about how my own ob-gyn had forbidden me from training for a mini-marathon when I was pregnant with Luna. There's a time and place. That's what we needed some of our most overweight patients to understand.

And wow, did they. They were so grateful to hear that message – not because they were lazy (they wouldn't have come to the clinic if they weren't eager and motivated to change their situations) but because the idea of *too* many lifestyle changes at once can be overwhelming, especially when you are tired, and hurting, and when just getting around the grocery store is daunting. A new way of eating *and* a whole new regimen of physical activity? Either one on its own is a lot; together, it can break you before you get started. I said the following so many times at conferences, group settings, everywhere, and it's worth repeating here: people who suffer from metabolic disease are not lazy. They have kids, they have grandkids, they work, they maintain relationships and families and households, they support the people around them, the list goes on. We have to be sensitive about the time and energy they are putting in to improve their health. The most common response to our "You don't need to exercise just yet" was some version of, "No, wait – are you serious?" Yes, we were. Because studies showed that exercise is *not* a good weight-loss strategy. (Some people will want to read that sentence again.) Are there benefits to exercise? Of course there are, both physical and mental. Yet even the American College of Sports Medicine attests that *exercise is not a good plan to lose weight*. On the other hand, it's probably a good way to help *keep* weight off, so exercise should be part of the long-term goal for everyone. We were focused on the food part.

In addition to the education about food choices, we also provided recipes. Brad and I experimented at home with new recipes and I shared them with patients, sometimes bringing in samples. I talked to proprietors of several local stores to encourage low-carb offerings, then passed on the information to our patients.

Brad and I also "produced" a series of videos that we called "Question and Answer Fridays," where I addressed questions I had received on my Facebook page and put on YouTube. Brad was the cameraman. Sometimes the sound quality wasn't great. The videos had titles like "How Carbs Become Fat," "What About Fruit on a LCHF Diet?" and "What Is Metabolic Syndrome?" These are still on YouTube. Search for "Fitter U."

Soon enough our patients and the team were experiencing amazing moments of shared triumph. On the walls of the clinic we posted Before and After photos, notes, pounds lost. We gave small rewards as patients reached weight loss milestones. They cheered for each other. One patient's insurance company actually contacted her to comment that they had noticed a dramatic decrease in her cholesterol level. Patti once said, "This is so rewarding. You see good things happening."

But something even more exciting was happening. Patients with diabetes were seeing their blood sugar levels drop and the need for diabetic medications decrease. We were pulling people off insulin at rates I could never have believed had I not been the physician taking care of them. I remember the first time we said about a patient, "Oh my god . . . that was the last of her insulin!"

To be honest, I was unprepared for such profound results with diabetes, and for it to happen so soon. *It rocked my world.* I was genuinely stunned by how quickly some of the significant positives occurred. The whole team was. I had read the literature published at that time, and knew that carbohydrate restriction could improve control of blood sugar and get people off meds. But in weeks? Sometimes in just *days*? We were pulling people off hundreds of units of insulin within weeks. Patient after patient was reversing – reversing, not merely managing – their way out of one of the world's most serious, consequential chronic diseases.

Their diabetes was going away. [16]

The speed may have surprised me, but the reversals made sense. Diabetes after all is a disease of elevated blood sugar, and blood sugar results primarily from breakdown of the carbohydrates we eat.

On the next page is my favorite nutrient diagram because it shows so clearly the reaction of blood sugar to each of the three macronutrients. Seeing the way blood sugar rises after consuming carbohydrates, a low-fat/high-carbohydrate diet makes no sense if you want to lower your blood sugar. But the reaction of blood sugar to fat consumption is basically flat. Energy for your body does not have to come from carbohydrates. Fat is a wonderful fuel source. Energy comes from fat consumed and *fat already stored* (think weight loss).

---

[16] It's important to note that their diabetes has been reversed, not cured. By sticking to the carbohydrate- restricted diet, they can maintain the reversal.

Because dietary fat does not have much of an insulin response, you have less of that fat-storage hormone hanging around.

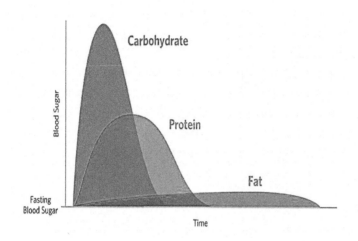

The diagram also shows how a well-formulated ketogenic diet cannot be "all protein," as it is sometimes negatively described (it should basically be very low-carb, moderate protein, and high-fat). Even though protein has a smaller effect on blood sugar than carbohydrates, it is still larger than fat.

~

Almost overnight the goal of our clinic focused more on diabetes than on weight management. Yet another pivot in my medical trajectory.

I was so happy to be doing so much deprescribing rather than prescribing.

Why isn't everyone doing what we're doing? I thought.

Given the suffering caused by diabetes, why is this common-sense approach still mostly a secret?

Where is this diet in the Dietary Guidelines?

WHAT IS GOING ON??

Not surprisingly, I got angry. Anger had driven me into medicine and would continue to guide my pivots. There was also an immediate aspect to address given that our patients' blood sugar levels were dropping significantly and quickly. While that was great, we had to adjust to this profound change – and with extreme care. We realized that our patients would need intense monitoring and instruction on managing their blood sugars and medications.

How would we do that?

~

I had learned so much in preparation for opening the clinic and I wasn't finished learning, not by a long shot. I tried always to be open-minded about what I didn't know, while confident about what I did.

I also felt it was vital that our team and I gather as much knowledge as possible because nutritional information was often passed on with notoriously scant scrutiny, compared to lots of other health-related information. The beliefs of nutritionists become the beliefs of the wider medical world. If medical schools provided evidence-based nutrition education to med students, who go on to communicate that information to their patients, we'd be in much better shape. But they don't. In a not-so-funny way, maybe it's a blessing that medical schools *don't* spend much time teaching nutrition, since they would end up passing on the same old status quo thinking about the supposed benefits of the low-fat, high-carb diet. Anyway, "nutrition education" at far too many medical schools is focused, curiously, *not* on what we eat. A majority of doctors receive fewer than twenty hours of nutrition training throughout their years of med school, most of which is spent discussing vitamins and vitamin deficiencies, something we seldom see in this country, or in-hospital tube and IV feeding. Their education does not cover the basic question of what to eat for specific diseases and risk factors.

WHAT IS GOING ON?

~ ~ ~

Chapter 9

What IS Going On?

What are the consequences for the lack of medical education about nutrition?

Without proper education, conventional wisdom and the status quo remain entrenched; dubious information is often communicated unthinkingly; and many doctors simply accept the findings of "the nutrition world," without checking for themselves whether the science is solid. The business model for so many doctors, as I had already discovered, revolved around prescribing medication for all kinds of conditions. I don't blame doctors (or most doctors, anyway) for this. It's the warped system that provides the incentive. The result is that certain supposed nutrition-related truths are simply regurgitated – e.g., this kind of dietary fat is bad; sodium intake should be lowered to extreme levels (another "fact" without evidence); "healthy" carbs are good for people with diabetes ("healthy" because they are high in micronutrients[17] and fiber, but too many carbs are too

---

[17] Micronutrients do not provide calories but are required for the body to function. Think vitamins and minerals. They are usually measured in small units, milligrams or micrograms.

many carbs). Soon enough, the public and the media all believe something to be true that isn't. They can even believe that something potentially harmful is helpful.

My original copy of Jeff Volek and Steve Phinney's *The Art and Science of Low Carbohydrate Living* was literally falling apart because I had read it and referred to it so often. But I had gone beyond their foundational text. The more I read, the more I came to see the sad – indeed tragic – truth. Much of the history behind the recommended American diet is downright ugly.

It will probably come as no surprise that the giant food and farming industries have a massive financial interest in how Americans eat. What I had *not* known, though, was that their influence over what we eat dates back to at least the 1930s, and that their power was (and remains) deep enough to make certain products more available and certain other products less so, regardless of the health benefits. Very often the more available food is far worse for us. The biggest food companies, then and now, often influenced the science being done, so that their products – among them, sugar, soda, vegetable oils, processed grains, food-like substances, and more – dominated the central aisles of the American supermarket. These massive companies funded self-validating nutrition studies and influenced nutrition departments across the country, including at our most prestigious and trusted institutions.

I want to make sure to acknowledge this: though I have contributed research to the fields of nutrition, obesity, and diabetes care, I did not myself do the hard, original research that uncovered the root problems around nutrition. Besides Steve Phinney and Jeff Volek, science journalists Gary Taubes and Nina Teicholz, to name two remarkable pioneers, each did intensive, years-long investigations into the science, pseudo-science, and politics behind Big Food and Big Medicine. What they brought to light in their books, Taubes' *Good Calories, Bad Calories* and *Why We Get Fat*, as well as Teicholz's *The Big Fat Surprise,* is remarkable. (If you haven't read these, put them on your must-read list now!) A great deal of the information in the following paragraphs, which I add for important background, comes from their research.

Take, for example, the old "food pyramid." We all know it. We were exposed to it when we were kids. It showed basic food groups and the number of servings healthy individuals should eat each day from each group, starting at the base with 6 to 11 servings of bread, cereal, rice and pasta – carbohydrates! At the top are fats and sugars, to be consumed sparingly. We were encouraged to follow the pyramid because supposedly we would be much likelier to live long, healthy lives.

In the end, the food pyramid did not show us how to eat for health.[18] It lacked *any evidence* that we were likelier to live healthy lives if we ate from those particular food groups, in those particular proportions.

---

[18] The Food Pyramid was replaced in 2011 by MyPlate which recommends a plate showing one-fourth each for fruits, vegetables, grains, and protein, with a "side" of (low-fat) dairy. Fats are not specifically listed, but MyPlate includes the recommendation that saturated fat should be limited. Following MyPlate recommendations will result in 200-300 grams of carbs for a person consuming 2000 calories a day.

No, the food pyramid ultimately gave rise to a much more troubling question: what happens if you give blanket nutritional advice to an entire country, and by default the entire globe, and the advice is based on either (a) no evidence or (b) incredibly weak evidence?

Take one massively important instance of dietary recommendations gone wild: the "diet-heart hypothesis." It argues that consumption of saturated fats leads to heart disease. The hypothesis really started gaining steam way back in the 1950s. Americans came to understand that dietary fat could kill you; that a high-fat diet, especially one with lots of saturated fat, was bad for you – raising your cholesterol, clogging your arteries, doing all kinds of bad stuff.

Except that a high-fat diet wasn't – and isn't – bad for you. The underlying science to this idea was flawed – indeed, manipulated – from the start. It's a fascinating, though deeply troubling, story.

With the growing prosperity of the post-World War II United States, an explanation was needed for changes in American bodies and health. Americans were starting to gain more weight. Heart disease was increasing. President Dwight Eisenhower, an athletic, generally healthy-looking man and military hero, suffered a heart attack in 1955 (which he survived), and something had to be blamed. The American public would be "comforted" by an explanation for the increasingly common, often fatal condition of coronary disease.

In the early 1950s, Ancel Keys, a physiologist at the University of Minnesota, started promoting the idea that the most likely cause of heart disease was a high-fat diet. He plotted statistics compiled by each of six countries, showing that death rates from heart disease were almost perfectly correlated with fat consumption, and he presented this data to various scientific audiences. But a 1957 paper, by two well-known statisticians working in public health, Jacob Yerushalmy and Herman Hilleboe, pointed out that data were actually available for *22* countries, not just six, and when all of these countries were included in the chart, the correlation between heart disease and fat consumption was far weaker. For example, people in countries like France and Switzerland ate a lot of fat, far more than we did in the US, but weren't dying at high rates from heart disease.

This evidence undermined Keys' theory, and he was not pleased. He responded by trying to prove his theory in a new study. In 1958 he launched the "Seven Countries Study," which, despite significant limitations, came to be among the most influential nutrition studies ever conducted.

In the Seven Countries Study, Keys wasn't just looking at national statistics as he had in the early 1950s. He was collecting his own data on diet and heart disease, from nearly 13,000 men in seven countries – mostly in Europe (Finland, Greece, Italy, Netherlands, and the former Yugoslavia) – but also in the US and Japan. By this point, Keys had shifted his idea to focus not so much on all fats but specifically on saturated fat and cholesterol as the culprits behind heart disease. Saturated fat and dietary cholesterol are most commonly found in eggs, dairy, shellfish, and meat – foods that human beings had been eating for millennia. Now, though, according to Keys, they were suspect. (He and others had conducted small preliminary experiments and found that saturated fats tended to raise total cholesterol.). The Seven Countries Study was the first multi-country study ever to observe and follow populations (called an "observational" study).

In 1970, Keys' landmark findings came out in a special publication by the American Heart Association (AHA).[19] For years, the AHA had embraced Keys' ideas about fats, even before his findings were published.[20] Keys' data now "proved" him correct – that consumption of saturated fats and dietary cholesterol were associated with higher rates of death from heart disease. The results seemed to validate Keys' hypothesis.

Except that they didn't.

There were many problems with the Seven Countries Study. For instance, it's fair to say that Keys cherry-picked his countries. He included only countries such as Italy and Greece where Keys knew, from his early investigations, that heart disease rates were low and people were eating very little saturated fat (largely due to the fact that their economies had been disrupted

---

[19] The Seven Countries Study also resulted in hundreds of publications, including eight books. sevencountriesstudy.com/study-findings/publications/

[20] In 1961, the AHA made recommendations that to prevent heart attacks people should minimize consumption of fats and foods with dietary cholesterol (such as eggs or shrimp). This advice was specifically aimed at people known to be at risk (family history, previous cardiovascular events). Over time it morphed into the AHA's recommendations for the general public, and was eventually adopted and enlarged by the *Dietary Guidelines for Americans*. Report by the Central Committee for Medical and Community Program of the American Heart Association. "Dietary fat and its relation to heart attacks and strokes." *Circulation.* Vol 23, Issue 1, 133-136. January 1961. www.ahajournals.org/doi/epdf/10.1161/01.CIR.23.1.133

by World War II, which affected what they ate, especially not a lot of meat). By contrast, Keys again did *not* include in his study countries such as France and Switzerland which, as researchers Yerushalmy and Hilleboe had pointed out, would contradict his hypothesis. This and many extraordinary details and flaws in the Seven Countries Study can be found in Teicholz's book, *The Big Fat Surprise*.

Ultimately, the problem with Keys' study is that it could show only an *association* between saturated fat and heart disease. It could not prove cause and effect; in other words, his data could never show that saturated fats *caused* heart disease. People who ate more saturated fats could also have been unhealthy in other ways: they may have exercised less or suffered more from war-time disruption. The nature of Keys' study could never discern, with any certainty, the exact cause of the health outcomes he observed. And he dismissed as unworthy of examination other possible dietary causes of heart disease; he was especially adamant that it could not be sugar.

Later, Alessandro Menotti, one of the original researchers in the Seven Countries study with Keys, re-analyzed the data using different categorizations of food and found that sweets and sugary desserts also correlated strongly with heart disease deaths. But Keys focused on saturated fats, and due to his charismatic, persuasive personality when promoting this idea, we are hobbled by this faulty theory to this day.

Back then, though, his theory was satisfying. It gave us something we believed we could now *control*, thus supposedly lowering the chance for heart attacks and related coronary disease and weight gain. Just eat less saturated fat! We could eat all the desserts and drink all the sodas we wanted, we just had to avoid the fats. Autopsies of people who died of heart disease showed fat in their arteries. Eat saturated fat, it will get in your arteries, you might eventually die of it, right? It made perfect sense. Eat saturated fat, it becomes fat in your blood. If A, then B. We had our culprit: dietary saturated fat.

Ancel Keys was on the cover of *Time* magazine in 1961. The impact of his study was huge, influencing dietary recommendations – particularly, the food pyramid – for decades, thus impacting the health and lives of tens of millions, arguably hundreds of millions. His theory was expanded upon by others who also decided that fat should be avoided, because fat was denser in calories than carbohydrates or protein. Avoid fat, eat a low-fat diet, eat a lot of carbohydrate-rich foods instead, and you'd be likely to lose weight. This was the thinking, even though in the 1970s, when this idea was adopted, no one had ever done an actual experiment on humans to find out if it was true. When they finally did do those studies – 30 years later, the same trials on low-fat/high-carb diets that informed my understanding when I started the IUH obesity clinic – it was clear that it wasn't true. All those conclusions and the dietary guidelines that went with them were horribly, tragically wrong. How damaging the mistake.

The advice about eating fat was the opposite of true. Recent rigorous "feeding studies" (a type of study where all the food that participants eat is provided by those conducting the study, thus encouraging adherence) have found that the levels of certain saturated fats in blood tend to *increase* on a low-fat/high-carbohydrate diet. The intake of saturated fat, if part of a well-formulated ketogenic diet, does not increase saturated fat in the blood; in fact, well-respected studies show that such a diet is strongly associated with *decreased* saturated fat in the blood! (Another sentence worth reading again.) This is critically important science. If people are to make informed choices about what they eat, they need to know what matters in their bodies, and that it matters which foods influence what. The status quo – *for decades*! – claimed that increased saturated fat levels in the blood were linked to increased risk for heart disease . . . yet it was all so wrong.

When I was working at a local hospital before I went to med school, a colleague of mine was so consumed by the anti-fat message that he obsessed over his fat intake to the point that he ate almost no fat. Instead, he ate bread, pizza crust, pasta, and other high-carb foods. Result? He was still overweight. Given the theories we'd all been taught, he was thoroughly perplexed. That's a data set of one, true, but the result remains unsurprising.

~

What is the human toll for this mistake, this bad science regarding fat? I hesitate to compare it to war or natural disaster. Yet in sheer numbers, in the amount of disease, misery, and ultimately death that this deceit caused and continues to cause, the impact is staggering. Millions and millions of people have been negatively affected by this misguided thinking and the institutional recommendations it spawned.

Look at diabetes alone. We had nowhere near the current incidence of this disease before low-fat/high-carb diets became standard. The prevalence of diabetes in the US increased almost 700% in the past sixty years, since Keys first showed up on the cover of *Time* – 700%! Today's statistics on diabetes are horrifying. About half the adults in this country have diabetes or prediabetes, and that doesn't include all those who have just insulin resistance or too much insulin; you can have elevated insulin levels for years, even decades, before your blood sugar rises and a diagnosis of prediabetes or diabetes is made. In a sense, elevated insulin levels essentially represent *pre*-prediabetes. Markers for diabetes might be normal during this period, but the body may be struggling to control blood sugar . . . until it can't. The health problems (comorbidities) often associated with diabetes – vision loss, kidney disease, nerve damage and, yes, even coronary artery disease – begin in this period when insulin levels rise to meet the challenge.

Every single day in the US, an average of 230 people has some body part amputated because of their diabetes.[21] One in three people with diabetes has kidney disease; diabetes is the leading cause of kidney failure

---

[21] "Each year, approximately 200,000 non-traumatic amputations occur. African Americans are 4 times more likely to experience diabetes-related amputation than whites. In the United States, every 17 seconds someone is diagnosed with diabetes, and every day 230 Americans with diabetes will suffer an amputation. . . . Throughout the world, it is estimated that every 30 seconds a leg is amputated. And 85% of these amputations were the result of a diabetic foot ulcer." Caffrey M. "Diabetic Amputations May Be Rising in the United States." *The American Journal of Managed Care.* December 13, 2018. ajmc.com/view/diabetic-amputations-may-be-rising-in-the-united-states

and the need for dialysis. Individuals with diabetes are at higher risk for developing certain cancers, especially of the liver and pancreas. And as we now know, diabetes is one of the most compromising pre-conditions in severe cases of Covid-19.

Is the institutionalized low-fat, high-carb diet responsible for *all* cases of type 2 diabetes? Of course not. But it's fair to say that it's responsible for a great deal of the spike. The circumstantial evidence is very strong. People have been convicted of crimes on less evidence.

I'm relying on solid circumstantial evidence for all foods where there's no strong clinical evidence for or against. That circumstantial evidence? Well, rates of obesity and diabetes in the US, as well as cardiovascular disease, took a sharp turn upwards soon after our government and major health organizations launched campaigns to cut down on fat, declared sugar to be a harmless, benign treat, and suggested that we all eat 6 to 11 servings of grains a day. Literally, they were recommending the equivalent of up to eleven slices of bread![22]

We now have a great deal of data showing that starches and sugars spike blood sugar, the key factor leading to diabetes. So that's some strong circumstantial evidence. We don't have a clinical trial to prove it, but doing that kind of trial, the kind that is likely to cause harm to participants – where some participants consume little starch and sugar and others consume a lot – would now be considered unethical.

---

[22] The current recommendation is 6 servings of grains a day, at least half whole grains.

~

Yes, conventional wisdom about the relationship between fat/saturated fat and heart disease was based on faulty or non-existent "evidence." What about other faulty conventional wisdom that tens of millions of people believe, and around which they organize their lives?

- *"To lose weight, eat less and exercise more."*

Wrong. Does it work? No. Who has tried it with lasting success? Answer: VERY few people. The culture and much of the medical establishment tell people it's all about calories in and calories out.

It's not.

And as I learned, while exercise provides lots (and lots) of benefits, weight loss isn't one of them. Yet people go to the gym and put in all kinds of time and effort. For most people, this will not contribute significantly to weight loss. (Weight maintenance? Probably.)

- *"If you diet, you will always feel hungry."*

False.

Reducing carbohydrates and increasing fats fill people up! They eat less without being told to do so. This has been shown in multiple studies. When patients say to me, "I can't live without bread/cake/peanut butter cups/fill-in-your own favorite," my first response is, "Spoken like someone who has never tried to live without bread/cake/peanut butter cups/fill-in-your own favorite." It's true! I said that to each patient who initially felt this way. The patient comment I heard most

101

consistently, after they tried carbohydrate restriction was, "I can't believe I'm not hungry" or " I can't believe I'm not craving x/y/z."

- **"You need carbohydrates to survive."**

No, you don't!

There has never been an absolute need for humans to consume carbohydrates. Even one of the pillars of the nutritional Status Quo, the USDA/"Institute of Medicine Dietary Reference Intakes Report," says so: "The lower limit of dietary carbohydrate compatible with life is apparently zero . . . " *Apparently zero*. Have you ever visited a friend at the hospital with a carbohydrate deficiency? No, because there is no such thing. There is no such thing as carbohydrate deficiency!

Personally, I would not want to live completely without carbohydrates, nor do I recommend that my patients totally give them up. Vegetables, for example, always have at least some carbs, but they are also a great source of micronutrients and fiber, and with butter or olive oil they're delicious and a good way to add fat. Just avoid the high-carb vegetables such as winter squash, carrots, potatoes, and sweet potatoes. I tell my patients, "No GPS – no grains, no potatoes, no sugar."

- **"A calorie is a calorie is a calorie."**

Misleading.

For the longest time, leading voices in the nutrition world taught us that a calorie is a calorie. But the low-carb concept, which represents a threat to the many authorities in the health and nutrition fields who have pushed what they've pushed for the past 60+ years, is predicated on the idea that not all calories are equal. So, 100 calories of sugar are not the same as 100 calories of kale or 100 calories of meat. This may seem obvious – each of these "packages" of 100 calories contain different amounts of both macro and micronutrients – but it goes against the American dietary gospel, which has long pushed Calories In, Calories Out, and argues that if you regularly exercise away the number of calories you consume, then you categorically cannot gain weight. The low-carb approach and all the compelling evidence supporting it are an affront to highly funded corporate strategies that push the low-fat, low-calorie, high-carb diet. It exposes a falsehood that was perpetrated decades ago, one used to sell Americans on a completely different diet, one that is less healthy and less filling, that makes us more prone to obesity and diabetes, and that makes so many people with issues around nutrition, diet, and health, generally, more miserable than they ever had to be.

In short, so much of the supposed science that formed the basis for the food pyramid – the USDA-recommended guidelines for how to eat healthy – was frankly baloney. Hypotheses that fat and cholesterol were bad for you were disproved decades ago. But food conglomerates and pharmaceutical conglomerates, aided and abetted by sometimes well-meaning bureaucrats at the USDA and FDA, had for so long stoked those false hypotheses that these ideas became institutionalized, never mind the absence of any hard evidence to support them. This institutionalizing, in turn, profoundly influenced the American diet and, in turn, American health outcomes.

But wait: Why, you might ask, would pharmaceutical companies root for a low-fat diet? Because it lowers your LDL cholesterol, while a low-carb diet has little effect on it (though a positive effect on nearly everything else).[23] If you have a multibillion-dollar business selling a drug that lowers your LDL cholesterol, then you need to keep your stories straight about what's good for you. And so the emphasis on lowering LDL – with a low-fat diet *and drugs*.

Later, in 2017, when some intrepid, science-supported researchers began to pipe up about the lack of evidence for the nexus between saturated fat and cholesterol, and between cholesterol (especially LDL) and cardiovascular diseases, the AHA doubled down, producing a statement about the dangers of saturated fat. Where did they get their data to support their theory? They cherry-picked them.[24] The statement largely ignored all existing science to the contrary, both "old" and recent. Not surprisingly, the statement neglected to mention that the AHA gets lots of money from giant food companies, including makers of refined vegetable oil. There is nothing remotely "whole food" or natural about refined vegetable oil. It's an industrial product: To turn seeds into oil form, they are bleached, and hexane is often used (stripped out after processing). It's lots of chemicals. It's crap. But vegetable oil *does* lower LDL cholesterol.

Your doctor either didn't tell you this or honestly doesn't know it: Changing your diet with the goal of lowering LDL cholesterol – the cholesterol type we're told to be most concerned about – is not associated with improved health outcomes. Not a single study out there

---

[23] LDL does go up for some people on a very low-carb (ketogenic) diet, at least temporarily. See the Glossary for details.

[24] Remember that the AHA was a huge supporter of Ancel Keys' diet-heart hypothesis and did not waver from that position for decades.

– zero, none – shows that a change in one's LDL cholesterol level, be it an increase or decrease, via dietary changes, will help you live a day longer. Simply put, while following a low-fat diet may decrease your LDL cholesterol, the next part we're led to believe – "therefore you do better" – has never been established. The "do better" part is assumed. In fact, zero evidence supports it.

Interestingly, one of the studies that the status quo, anti-saturated fat advocates like to cite – the Mediterranean diet study – found a decrease in secondary cardiovascular disease (CVD) events[25] and in mortality for consumers of a Mediterranean diet compared to those on a standard diet. Yet there were no differences in the LDL cholesterol levels between the two groups.[26] *Hmmm* . . . CVD events and mortality down for one group; LDL, no difference between the groups. Hmmm indeed. To me, and to anyone who looks at the results with a scientific eye, that sounds like no correlation between LDL and CVD. LDL is not the predictor of CVD that we (or perhaps better, they) have been espousing. And that's just one of many studies that suggests we need to rethink our focus on (obsession with?) LDL cholesterol as a major coronary risk factor.

More and more I understood the clear, scientific reasons that diets failed when they were based on these simple, supposedly intuitive bumper stickers:

---

[25] Secondary CVD occurrences are subsequent to an earlier heart attack.

[26] The first group was on a "Mediterranean-type diet" and the other group consumed "a prudent Western-type diet."

Fat = Mostly Bad
Saturated Fat = Always Bad
To Stay Thin, Limit Your Calories & Work Out

To repeat: dietary fat isn't nearly the problem that so many doctors, nutritionists, national health organizations, and the government told us it was. Meanwhile, something else in our diet that we *can* control – carbohydrates – *is* a problem. And remains a problem. Quite likely, *the* problem.

Decades of flawed recommendations had been perpetrated on anyone who ate food. Especially Americans. For generations. For more than a half century, we've been encouraged to eat the wrong things.

Status quo thinking is killing us. I don't believe I'm being melodramatic. I believe I've shown how status quo thinking, built on wildly erroneous thinking, harms us. It has harmed those who came before and, unless we expose it, will harm those to come. We have to replace it with evidence-based thinking and guidelines that actually help people.

Exposing erroneous thinking is the first step in the process.

~   ~   ~

Chapter 10

What IS Going On? Part 2

A particular passion of mine as doctor and patient advocate has been investigating how status quo thinking affects our health. With many of the patients I saw – and millions and millions like them – status quo thinking often perpetuates health inequities. Sadly, there are countless examples of health inequity happening every day in this country, resulting in health outcomes that are worse for some than for others. It's important that the public and the "system" understand this, because no one should be treated this way, with less access than others to decent health care.

The status quo isn't a problem merely because it's the status quo – that is, because it resists change. It's a problem because it resists changing a system that leaves much to be desired and can be so much better. It's a problem because entrenched forces make positive change harder than it ought to be.

I had no illusions that our work in nutrition, obesity, and diabetes care was the linchpin to overhauling the entire American healthcare system. (Though I could dream . . .) My sincere hope was that, via a transparent, evidence-based explanation of what the foods we eat do to us, and through relentless promotion of that explanation to the general public, we might sidestep some traditional channels and tip the scales a little bit back in favor of the individual, whether she's a poor single mom or anyone else. With knowledge comes power. With knowledge comes choice. My hope was that our work would allow individuals to take better care of themselves, mostly through diet.

No one ever said it would be easy.

One of the "traditional channels" that determined our eating and health, the Dietary Guidelines for Americans, turned out to be bad for the public's health overall. They were based on bad methodology and therefore bad science, influenced by Big Food.[27] In turn, the Guidelines drove our perception of what Big Food provides and our apparently essential need for those products.

An example: the Guidelines dictate what's served for school breakfasts and lunches, including donuts, fruit juice, and chocolate or strawberry milk. (Donuts?! Think elevated blood sugar, then the crash around mid-morning, during math class.) Milk served for these meals cannot be more than 1% fat. Fat is still seen as a bigger menace than sugar. And everyone gets the same food, whether you're a tiny, skinny third-grader or an obese fifth-grader. How can that be? They need different foods! Their bodies are clearly different. The foods that are going to be most healthy for each of them will, to a meaningful extent, differ. Technically, the fifth-grader with obesity falls outside the boundaries of the guidelines, which are, after all, supposed to be

---

[27] By Big Food, I mean, well, all those giant producers and distributors of so much of the food that we consume, from Procter & Gamble, Cargill, and ADM to Frito-Lay, Coca-Cola, McDonald's, Burger King, and on and on.

aimed solely at "healthy individuals." But never mind (apparently) that this fifth-grader is not healthy. He will get the same breakfast and lunch as those with very different nutritional needs. What he eats is set for him by dietary guidelines that don't apply to him. Why? The mandate for the Guidelines is to keep Americans healthy. Is the following logical to you?

The Guidelines say they are for all healthy Americans. But who are these healthy Americans?

(a) About 50% of the adults in this country have diabetes or prediabetes.
(b) 88% of adults are not in optimal metabolic health (*eighty-eight percent!*).[28]
(c) Which means the greatest possible percentage of the adult population that the Guidelines could apply to is a paltry 12%.
(d) Which means the Guidelines, appropriate for only a tiny sliver of the US adult population, most affect those for whom the guidance is inappropriate, especially people with metabolic diseases.

In addition to the healthy/not healthy discrepancy, the Guidelines fail to account for different dietary needs or circumstances of lower socioeconomic

---

[28] Meaning they have abnormal markers for one or more: blood pressure, blood sugar (fasting glucose, A1c), triglycerides, HDL, waist circumference. If a person has three or more of these markers, he or she has metabolic syndrome (See the Glossary). Araujo J, Cai J, Stevens J. "Prevalence of Optimal Metabolic Health in American Adults: National Health and Nutrition Examination Survey 2009-2016." *Metabolic Syndrome and Related Disorders.* 2019 Feb;17(1):46-52. liebertpub.com/doi/10.1089/met.2018.0105

status and ethnic/racial minorities, who comprise a disproportionate part of the 88% for whom the guidelines do not apply.

A report from the Food4Health Alliance found that of the 56 reviews of dietary evidence that were undertaken by the 2020 Dietary Guidelines Advisory Committee, over 90% were severely compromised because they neglected to account for race/ethnicity or socioeconomic status, or they used samples that could not be generalized and applied to the greater US population. Despite this, the Guidelines clearly state that this policy is intended for all Americans, regardless of race, ethnicity, or socioeconomic status.

The Guidelines did not account for, say, an eleven-year-old boy who attends public school in a large city, lives with his mother and three-year-old sister, and whose family rarely has enough money for the groceries they need. The boy is already overweight. He eats his breakfast and lunch at school, where he is provided with grains, juice, low-fat chocolate milk, processed foods and processed meats; if he's lucky, he'll have a small bag of carrots. He has difficulty concentrating in school.

When the boy gets home he's hungry, so he searches the apartment for food. Most times he grabs a piece of bread – one of the foods that's consistently around – and orange juice (high in sugar, like all fruit juices) or more low-fat milk. For dinner, the boy's mom makes something she got through the Special Supplemental Nutrition Program for Women, Infants, and Children (WIC).[29] Maybe tonight he gets lucky and

---

[29] When his sister turns five they will no longer be eligible for WIC.

it's chicken and noodles, with a banana for dessert.

The Guidelines are revised every five years. What will the next revision do to help this boy stay healthy? We don't know – but until then, he'll be getting steadily sicker. He already has many struggles ahead of him. He's starting off in a tough spot. He is tired, obese, and all around unhealthy.

Do we as a society blame this boy for his situation at age 11?

Sadly, we do it all the time.

If only he listened to what his doctor told him to eat.

He's just lazy and has no self-control.

He just needs to exercise more.

His parents are asleep at the wheel.

None of these, as you can see from his story, is true or fair. America, and the forces of greed and expedience and resistance to change, did this to the boy. The system ignored the needs of a child who can't make his own choices. Or, more accurately, his available choices are all pretty bad ones. This is not a lazy child, but a child whose mother can't afford to put on the table what she would really like to feed him. How can we keep doing this to the most vulnerable?

Health inequity stinks. The inherent racism and economic elitism in the Guidelines and so much of our healthcare system stink. This has all been happening right under our noses. It's been going on for decades. We tend not to talk much about food when it comes to health inequity. When we do, it's limited to the issue of food access. That needs to be addressed, of course, but fixing access alone will not fix the larger problem. Not long ago our newspaper printed a feel-good story about local kids who had donated over a thousand boxes of cereal to the food bank. As I looked at the accompanying picture of sugared everything, I could not help but shudder.

When will we wake up?

~

Over the years there have been many brave dissenters, scientific researchers with integrity, who pushed back against "conventional wisdom." They understood that the data couldn't possibly support the low-fat theory. What happened to these voices? In many cases, their careers were ruined by Big Nutrition. One nutritionist and physiologist from Britain, John Yudkin, a pioneer of the low-carb diet, who was doing research in the 1960s, believed there was another culprit, or at least a more direct culprit, behind heart disease and bad health outcomes. It wasn't dietary fat. It was sugar, which at the time had exploded in the American diet.

Remember Ancel Keys, author of the Seven Countries Study and the man who landed on the cover of *Time*? He attacked Yudkin's reputation, ridiculing him. Keys not only buried people who contradicted him, he did his best to bury any science that contradicted him. Keys was one of the lead investigators on the longest, most rigorous tests of his hypothesis ever conducted, called the Minnesota Coronary Survey (MCS, sometimes referred to as the Minnesota Coronary Experiment or MCE), funded by the U S Public Health Service and the National Heart Institute. Launched in 1968, MCS was not an "observational" study, like the one he had done in Seven Countries. That study, remember, could not generate the kind of reliable, cause-and-effect data that establishes hard evidence for an idea. Only a more rigorous *clinical* trial can do that. MCS was such a clinical trial. It was enormous, with more than 9,000 subjects; it included both men and women, which was unusual since nearly all studies until that time had been conducted on men only; and it lasted an extremely long time for a clinical trial, an impressive four and a half years.

There was another reason this trial was extraordinary: the subjects all lived in mental hospitals or a nursing home, meaning their food selection could be controlled. The Minnesota researchers designed the menus and knew what the participants were eating. The type of data gleaned from such a regimented study is far more reliable than data from people who self-report their food intake on questionnaires. Studies have shown repeatedly that people can't remember what they eat or simply lie. The MCS gave half the population a diet with 18% saturated fat – which was considered a normal percentage at the time but roughly double what Americans now consume – while the other half of the study population was fed 9% saturated fat, with the remaining fat provided by milk, cheese, and meat all modified with corn oil, plus corn oil for cooking, and soft corn oil margarine. All the special food was manufactured – surprise! – by industry to help with the experiment. MCS was an extraordinary undertaking, with great promise of providing definitive data on Keys' diet-heart hypothesis.

It didn't turn out the way the investigators expected.

Saturated fat was not found to increase the risk of dying from heart disease. If anything, the saturated fat-rich diet kept patients in the study healthier than the corn oil version. So what happened when the results of this paradigm-shifting study were published?

Nothing. For sixteen years after the study's completion, those who conducted it did not publish their results – and even then, in 1989, the chosen journal was an obscure, little-read publication, almost guaranteed to attract little notice. The massive study, costing taxpayers millions of dollars, was ignored, because its results challenged "findings" that Big Food and the Establishment nutrition community were so invested in. The study's results got buried – almost literally – and it wasn't even that hard to do. Data from the study languished for decades in the basement of the study's principal investigator, Ivan Frantz, Jr.,[30] until an NIH researcher tracked down Frantz's son, who said he hadn't cleared out his father's basement, then looked and found magnetic tapes and punch cards (!) with the trial data. When the NIH investigator, Christopher Ramsden, re-analyzed the data from this randomized controlled trial (that part's good), he concluded that saturated fat had no proven negative effect. An even more stunning finding to emerge from those original computer tapes: For the older MCS men and women, the more they lowered their cholesterol, the *more* likely they were to die of a heart attack.

It would have been nice to think that the AHA, perceived as the unbiased leader in the field of heart disease research, treatment, and prevention, would have admitted their mistake. Of course they didn't. That's not how these organizations work. But what they have

---

[30] Ancel Keys was another major investigator.

done, as I'll discuss, is slowly accept (in the fine print in their recommendations) that the high-fat foods they used to insist were unhealthy might not be. But by keeping this in the fine print, no major changes get made and doctors and dietitians continue to believe what they've always believed.

There is lots of good, groundbreaking, status quo-overturning scientific research going on in the area of nutrition. But I came to understand that a lot of nutritionists serve on important panels and are compensated to do so; many of these panels decide what constitutes a healthy diet, which in turn gets used by organizations like the American Medical Association, the American Heart Association, the American Diabetes Association, and others to provide guidelines for a "healthy diet." There are potential conflicts all over the place. And when you've believed something all your career, it becomes difficult to accept new evidence, especially when that evidence points to behavior you have always seen as harmful.

All my reading and clinical work and my own research led me to this painful conclusion: In the world of nutrition science, evidence is often inconvenient for those dedicated to defending the status quo. Thus, it gets ignored or even maligned, along with the author(s). Some authorities are just unwilling to change their minds, or simply have too much invested – reputationally, financially, psychologically – to wake up.

The status quo keeps on status quoing.

~ ~ ~

Chapter 11

Anger Rising

Crying happens a lot in medicine, and a lot in the field of obesity care. But most of the crying I witnessed from patients getting emotional at the weight-loss clinic was not for sadness. Nor was it for joy.

It was for rage. Disbelieving rage.

Why didn't someone tell me this before?

You mean, I could've saved myself from bypass surgery?

I never had to go on insulin?

Wow! Nobody, nobody really helped me like this before.

No one ever told me what to eat – just to exercise and lose weight.

Many of my patients, exposed to evidence-based explanations for how various components of food work on the body, realized, sometimes bitterly at first, that they had missed a huge opportunity to do something about their health much sooner *if only someone had told them*. If only vital nutritional/behavioral information that could have made a profound difference in their lives had not been kept from them. While these patients were grateful for the help we at the clinic were now providing, they had their moments of *God, none of this*

116

had to happen to me . . . it was all preventable! What made their anger sometimes burn even more was the realization that the medical environment *still* had not seen the light, *still* largely advocated the less effective, less proven (or unproven, or disproven), often more harmful "solution." Patients told me how furious it made them to go from our clinic to an appointment at another doctor's office, and while sitting in that waiting room, the TV would be tuned to some pharma-sponsored "health" channel, pushing the benefits of a low-fat, carb-heavy diet, along, of course, with the diabetes meds to help along the way. And then their own doctors would *still* tell them some version of, "If you just got up and exercised, that would really turn things around."

We knew we still had a big fight in front of us, but the staff and I were committed to educating everyone we could.

Early on, my boss, Al Gatmaitan, the CEO of our region of IUH and a huge champion of our weight-loss program from the start, asked, "Sarah, it's great that you're getting these results. Now, how do we scale it?"

I spent a long time trying to answer that question.

We had big dreams. We set firm goals. We wanted to transform the whole state of Indiana. I became part of our hospital's Ambulatory Quality Committee, and pushed to make it mandatory that low-carbohydrate be presented as a dietary option to everyone with metabolic disease who came through the system. The resolution passed unanimously, the first of its kind (at least that my staff and I could unearth) by any healthcare system in the country.

That was a good start. But I still couldn't figure

out an answer to my boss's excellent, basic question: how could we scale it?

~

The question morphed into an obsession. It was great that we were helping hundreds of obese, insulin-resistant and/or diabetic patients in Indiana, and some from surrounding midwestern states. But what about the millions and millions of people around the country and the world? Al, my very supportive boss, was recruited for a more senior position in the IUH statewide organization, so he was no longer overseeing me.

Now it was my team and me versus a less supportive administration. That's when a new problem emerged. I started feeling pressure from the higher-ups that the clinic was not making enough money.

"Are you kidding me?" I snapped at a new administrator. "Do you have any idea how much money we save our patients? Their families? Their employers?"

"You say that," he said, "but can you prove it?" He threatened staff cuts.

Once again, anger fueled me. The instant that conversation ended, I phoned the nutrition department at Purdue University, introduced myself to the person who answered, and announced, "I'm interested in finding a researcher who wants to compare the benefits of our weight-loss department versus standard of care." I paused. "I should mention that I have no funding for this project. I mean, zero dollars."

Amazingly, one of Purdue's researchers *was* interested in conducting a pilot study. He came to our office, selected at random 50 of our patients with

118

diabetes, and set out to compare them to 50 patients being treated with the standard diabetes management program by educators at IUH, so they all came from the same system. Guess what? (I bet you can, by now.) Our small, unfunded project showed that our patients enjoyed the same or, truth be told, better metabolic results on a low-carbohydrate diet, while also enjoying significant cost savings versus the current conventional way of treating diabetes and obesity. While the study did not get written up as a full paper (that was never my primary intention), it was presented at a conference of the National Lipid Association in 2015 and served its purpose: validating our clinic and proving that we were not just effective but also economically viable, should anyone question that again.

~   ~   ~

Chapter 12

Getting There

As carefully as we explained the science of nutrition and human physiology to our patients, it was a lot to take in. Often they asked us to clarify the differences among the major dietary approaches, and how they fit in with our weight-loss approach.

The whole-food, low-carb diet: When people eat low-carb (under 130 grams a day; some recommend 100), they eat less. Studies show that caloric consumption goes down by approximately 20%, despite the fact that your diet consists of a greater percentage of fat, which has a higher calorie density. Fat has nine calories per gram; carbs and protein each have four. Why would eating more fat make you eat less? Because fat makes you feel full. You eat less *because you don't feel like eating more*, a much more effective way to "manage" your eating than the failed, miserable, generations-old strategy of trying to eat less by telling yourself to eat less.

Eating a low-carb, higher-fat diet removes the deprivation aspect. The healthiest instructions about eating – eat when you're hungry; eat until you feel full – are the instructions we gave our patients. And it generally worked because it was scientifically, physiologically sound. There is nothing scientifically sound in telling people whose bodies are biologically craving some food to simply just not follow their craving.

For our patients, not having to count calories was thrilling and freeing.

The ketogenic diet: This is a very low-carb diet – to the max, if you will. Depending on one's goals and metabolic health, the cutoff for carbohydrates can be 50 grams a day, or 30, or even 20. If you have diabetes and you're interested in reversing it, a well-formulated ketogenic diet can work. If you no longer produce insulin, you can dramatically reduce the amount of insulin therapy you need; for patients with type 2 diabetes who are still making insulin, the goal of getting completely off insulin therapy is absolutely reasonable for most people. Once your weight or insulin goals are reached and you've been stable for a while, you may be able to increase carb consumption, *carefully*.

The vegetarian diet: Great! You can get adequate high-quality protein with nuts and dairy. If you're willing to add fish (which makes this a pescatarian diet), even better. Fresh vegetables are great; fresh fruit, in moderation, can be good, but because of fruit's high sugar content, my patient population had to be careful. Eating fruit can raise blood sugar and insulin tremendously. Our program required five servings of non-starchy vegetables per day, while discouraging most fruit. Small quantities of berries are fine and they're especially good with heavy cream. Plus, you get an extra "shot" of fat!

The vegan diet: Vegans do not eat any animal products, including dairy. If you have never had exposure to large amounts of sugar and refined carbohydrates (which is true of almost no one these days), and you've maintained a good weight on a vegan diet, and you're very careful with what kind of foods you select (without animal products, you must take care to get enough protein and micronutrients): more power to you – continue with the vegan diet.

Unfortunately, few people on a vegan diet are on a *whole food* vegan diet. Vegans argue that their diet is so full of fiber that it keeps them full longer, so they can restrict calories. But you can follow a vegan diet and still eat potato chips too much of the time. The vegan diet, as it's often practiced, may not provide sufficient nutrients, meaning many people have to supplement. Vegans must be incredibly selective; because of their choices, their diet very often tends to be very high-carb, low-protein – which is my particular concern about a vegan diet in kids. In fact, the Royal Academy of Medicine in Belgium considers a vegan diet for children "unethical" and potentially dangerous unless there is medical supervision.

The Mediterranean diet: This diet originated in the countries bordering the Mediterranean Sea, but has come to be associated especially with Greece and Italy. Embraced by Ancel Keys in the 1960s, it has been "labeled" and promoted as a healthy diet since the 1980s. There are many versions of the Mediterranean diet, which makes it difficult to assess, but usually it emphasizes whole grains, fruits, legumes – all high in carbs – and vegetables; in lesser amounts, dairy products, fish, and poultry/eggs; small amounts of sugar; and occasional lean red meat. Olive oil is the main fat, and there can be lots of it. Although the typical Mediterranean diet is not low-carb, it is usually lower than the standard American diet, features less processed food, and can be modified to fit a carbohydrate-restricted lifestyle.

A diet with meat: Meat is good for people. It's an important source of nutrients. What's insane right now isn't the meat itself but the way we provide it – via "factory farming," which herds large numbers of animals together, often confined indoors their entire lives. They are usually dosed with hormones and antibiotics. When people look back on this time period, factory farming is one of those practices about which they'll say, "How in the world could they have done that? What were they thinking?" We *know* it's bad for the Earth; we don't think, we know. It's cruel to the animals. If we let animals pasture, and eliminate all the soy and corn crap they are fed, we wouldn't require all the pesticides and chemical fertilizers because we would have natural fertilizer. We could get away from monoculture (growing only a single plant species in a given field, which depletes the soil of nutrients needed for fertility and increases the spread of plant and insect disease). We could go back to rotating crops. In fact, pasturing beef cattle has been shown to *decrease* CO_2. True, it doesn't make up for the increase in methane they produce, but it sequesters CO_2 in the ground rather than putting it in the atmosphere. Still, we need to massively change some of our farming practices. Listen to farmers who take seriously the health of their animals and the environment. This kind of agriculture is known as regenerative farming, and there's plenty to read on it, written by both farmers and animal science experts. Bottom line: don't bash the meat or a diet that includes meat; bash factory farming.

~

If you look at cultures around the world, you see that humans can exist well on a spectrum of dietary intakes, so long as it's mainly a whole food-based diet. Some cultures eat mostly plant-based foods (or are vegetarian, as are many people in India) and have low levels of heart disease and cancer. As Steve Phinney and Jeff Volek pointed out in their book, the Masai in Africa and the Inuit in the Arctic consumed very few carbs, a diet that's roughly 75-85% fat, and they did great, also having low levels of heart disease and cancer. Humans can exist and thrive on both ends of the spectrum *until you add sugar and processed foods and you overload on carbohydrates and artificial ingredients.*

We've gone wrong with our diet for a really long time. But it's not because of the saturated fat we're eating or the animal products. It's the carb-rich processed foods.

Enough.

~

In 2015, our already great clinic staff expanded by two valuable, full-time members. Amanda Dehne had been an RN in cardiology. She decided to start in her new role as a nurse practitioner for "a while" at the obesity clinic, and got drawn to it. She's still there, lucky for our patients. Tamara Hazbun, family doctor and invaluable friend, had grown frustrated with family medicine. Many of her patients had diabetes, prediabetes or obesity, yet she had no time to address these situations one-on-one, no opportunity to address their problems at a root level. It was the same frustration I had felt in primary care. She began referring her patients to us because of our success with low-carb, whole food (sometimes ketogenic) diets, supported by frequent monitoring.

Eventually Tamara reached the same breaking point that I had. She wanted to go beyond just referring patients to us; she considered practicing with us. I was thrilled at the prospect. She wanted to be part of a saner, more evidence-based approach to getting people healthier, or at least less sick. Our "radical" aim was not simply to manage chronic illness, which had become essentially the dictionary definition of primary care medicine. Our protocol was designed to teach and inform patients, in the belief that they understood more than most doctors assumed they could. It's sad to say but the typical setting for American family medicine is not geared for teaching or learning, by patients *or* physicians.

Tamara couldn't switch right away because she had a whole panel of family medicine patients she was responsible for. You can't just drop patients. It takes a while to ensure that they're properly transferred to another provider. In the meantime, she signed up for the coursework she needed for board certification in obesity medicine. She started coming over to our clinic to see patients a few hours a week. She passed her obesity boards and spent more time with us, while gradually reducing her primary care practice workload. Within a year, she had moved over to the clinic full time.

Tamara wasn't just a valuable addition to our medical staff. She was also an asset in our bureaucratic battles (less belligerent than you-know-who). At one point, for some reason, the administration decided to make cuts to our program – or, rather, they wanted us to charge patients more. I pointed out that that would keep away many people in need of our services. After some back and forth, they relented. They wouldn't force the change.

I don't know if it was the letter Tamara wrote to them pointing out that by upping the charge, the administration could be accused of bias, since the people they were targeting for the new charge were almost all overweight or obese. Not that *we* were accusing the administration of that, mind you . . . just that, you know, people might look at it that way.

I don't know if my at times pugnacious reputation preceded me and they decided they didn't want to fight me on this.

Either way, fine.

~

I felt the need to do more. I started writing a grant proposal seeking NIH funding for a low-carb study. But the more people I spoke with, the more of a fool's errand it appeared to be. I grew skeptical about getting approved. At obesity and nutrition conferences, other researchers kept telling me that I would never get funding for such a study. Doctors and scientists far more prominent and widely published than I had pursued the same idea – studying the science, safety, and efficacy of low-carb – and they'd been turned down repeatedly.

"The NIH won't fund a low-carb study," one colleague told me bluntly, "because they think people can't stick to it."

It was yet another disappointing instance of an institution supporting pure dogma.

We won't fund research for a low-carb study because people won't follow that diet; they won't follow the diet because there's no data to support it; ergo, we won't fund such a study.

It was lame-brained reasoning at its circular worst. But if Big Medicine really thought that way, then how could I *ever* get funding? I would have to find another way.

And then, amazingly, the other way happened, with alarming speed and generosity, as if the stars had aligned.

~   ~   ~

Chapter 13

Stars Align

I was invited to give a TEDx talk in May 2015, hosted at Purdue University. The title of my proposed speech: "Reversing Type 2 Diabetes Starts with Ignoring the Guidelines."

Everyone's response?

Umm . . . no.

It wasn't the subject matter that was the problem. It was the title. One of my friends said it was "too long, too messy, and won't get any attention."

Ever headstrong, I decided I would not change it.

Because why? The title stated clearly what the talk was about. It addressed the epidemic in medicine: status quo thinking. It didn't seem right to come up with something "catchier" but less accurate. (Anyway, *I* thought it was catchy.) And since I believed that one of medicine's biggest problems was doctors underestimating the ability of mere mortals to grasp basic scientific concepts, I wasn't inclined to dumb things down now.

(Then again, my issue had been with the way we underestimate the ability of *patients* – not doctors – to understand science. This time, I'd be speaking mostly to non-medical professionals. Maybe a catchier title was needed.)

The instructions for a TEDx presentation are strict – 18 minutes, memorized, no cue cards – but I was not particularly nervous. After all, I'd given a version of the talk countless times over the previous several years. One of my major points, as you know by now, was that we needed to eat more dietary fat. Yet that fairly simple bit of advice confused lots of new listeners because they didn't want to *be* fat. They wanted less body fat so why was I advocating eating more fat? The problem was largely, maybe even fatally, semantic. I included a line in the speech about how it might make things so much easier "if we just called dietary fat something else, like rainbows and butterflies."

As the date for the speech neared, I rehearsed my talk in front of Tamara, and then Tamara and her husband Tony Hazbun, a professor of molecular biology in Purdue's College of Pharmacy. Though writing the material came naturally and I was comfortable in front of an audience, I needed to practice the speech many times to commit it to memory and keep it to the assigned time limit.

Tamara said she loved it but for one thing – she hated the line about rainbows and butterflies. It was stupid.

I kept it in.

I rehearsed the speech for two other esteemed colleagues, Dr. Eric Westman, the co-founder and director of the Duke Keto Medicine Clinic, and Jacqueline Eberstein, former nurse for Dr. Atkins, he of the famous diet. When I finished the speech, Jackie said she liked it but for one part.

"What was that about rainbows and butterflies?" she wondered. "It doesn't make any sense."

I gave in. I took the line out. (I still think it works.)

A few days before TEDx, I had another speaking engagement, addressing a gathering of a national physicians group for obesity care at the Obesity Medicine Association conference in Denver. Tamara and I attended the event together.

Though comfortable with public speaking, I didn't feel particularly outgoing. That probably comes as a surprise to you. Few people who know me would call me an introvert, yet I often feel like one. I like people but I don't always enjoy talking to new folks. The obesity conference felt like a perfect opportunity to make more of an effort. As Tamara and I settled into our shared hotel room, I told her, "For the next two days, I'm going to force myself to talk to people." She laughed, to think that I thought shyness and an unwillingness to engage were my issues.

But maybe it was that resolve that led to the next giant pivot in my life. Maybe it was just karma. I gathered the nerve to approach one of the stars of the Denver conference and our whole field, Steve Phinney, co-author of *The Art and Science of Low Carbohydrate Living*, the book that I had read and reread and reread. He was the godfather of low-carb research and had become one of my heroes in the world of nutrition and health, having fought the fight since the late 1970s. He had been in academia decades before, but left that world partly because he was frustrated by the difficulty of getting grant funding for research projects. I could relate. For years, Steve's was a voice in the wilderness. Then he connected with his future co-author, Jeff Volek, at the time a young researcher at the University of Connecticut, and together they published dozens of papers, with scientific support for the benefits of low-carb. But they knew they had to do even more studies – to be taken seriously, to get attention, not to be dismissed. To have the ammunition to show just how wrong the status quo thinking was in nutrition. Along with others, Steve and Jeff ran clinical trials on low-carb (in both metabolically healthy and sick populations), saturated fat, ketosis,[31] and more.

When I spotted Steve at the obesity conference, I replayed in my head the vow I'd made to myself and Tamara, and approached him. He was talking to a small group of conference attendees but I didn't care. I went right up and tapped him on the shoulder. After breathlessly introducing myself, I said, "Steve, we have to talk."

He looked at me with curiosity. "Okay," he said.

"I've read your books. I read the science and it all makes sense. I've been using your diet and lifestyle approach in my clinic, and it has had dramatic effects on my patients. But we've got a problem with LDL cholesterol. It rises in some people, even though they seem to be healthy and I don't understand why. We need to understand the change more to ensure we're doing the right thing for patients. Can I tell you what we're doing in Indiana?" I didn't bother to wait for an answer, and proceeded to document our progress.

He listened intently. When I finally took a breath, he said, "Funny, we're doing the same thing." Then he asked me a hundred questions. I had a million of my own for him. The conversation shifted to the current economics of diabetes treatment, more as something to

---

[31] In ketosis, your body is primarily using fat, not carbohydrates, as its main energy source. See the Glossary for details.

be "managed" than halted or reversed. I had long thought that one effective approach would be to involve employers because a) it's really expensive for them (along with the affected individuals) to pay the health insurance for this illness, including the monthly medicines and b) companies lose countless employee-days to the sickness.

At some point, Steve raised an eyebrow.

"Oh, my goodness," he said. "Can I take you to dinner?"

Of course I said yes. Tamara joined us for the dinner that changed the trajectory of my professional life.

Over a two-and-a-half-hour dinner at a local restaurant, where Steve, Tamara, and I dined on wine, delicious buffalo steak, and asparagus in bleu cheese and butter, more than once I found myself thinking, *My god, I'm eating dinner with Steve Phinney*! Steve Phinney, who had been on a quest to understand the pluses and minuses of low-carb nutrition since 1975!

I told him more about what we were doing at our clinic. I told him that we had a waiting list hundreds of names long.

At some point during the meal, Steve said, "We're starting a company. We have the funding. Basically, we're trying to implement what you're talking about. We're looking for a site to do a low-carbohydrate ketogenic diet study. Sarah, it sounds like you're the physician who should oversee it. You'll be the principal investigator. Can we do it at IUH?"

Are you serious?

By the time dinner ended and we returned to the hotel, plans were in place to fund a large clinical trial out of my department at IUH Arnett. This development was stunning, bizarre, amazing – almost too good to be true. I could stop writing grant proposals. I could stop worrying about NIH headaches. I felt some chagrin because Tamara's husband Tony had worked his butt off for his NIH grants, often waiting years to get his projects green-lit. And I was experiencing the upside-down of that, a thrilling rarity: *Here's some money . . . Ready . . . Go!* I had to pinch myself.

In the hotel elevator, Tamara and I exited at our floor. Before the doors closed, we said goodnight to Steve, my new research partner. Tamara and I were flying back home the next morning and Steve wished me luck on my next speech, sort of.

"You better be good, Sarah," he said, smiling. "The average TEDx talk gets fifty thousand views." I was okay if I got just a thousand.

When I got to our hotel room, I texted Brad and my mom.

Life changing dinner tonight. Nothing will be the same.

~   ~   ~

Chapter 14

Virta

When I woke the next morning I had to think for a moment. *Did that really happen?*

I flew home, excited as always to see my family, and psyched to give my TEDx talk. I knew how much Brad and the kids wanted to attend but it conflicted with a youth soccer tournament, and both Noah's team and Ava's were playing. At least I would have Mom and my clinic staff in the audience. There had been some buzz leading up to the talk, thanks to the passionate "low-carb community."

There were eight TEDx speakers that day: four before the break, four after. I was delighted when they told me I would speak second. I could get it over with and relax for the other presentations.

When the first speaker finished (a South American filmmaker), I took the stage, confident in my message. At this point, it was almost impossible for me to feel nervous talking about these topics because I knew the material so well. If I skipped over a point or found myself exploring a side road I thought my listeners might appreciate, I could always find the way back.

Still, a TEDx talk is different. It's memorized and eighteen minutes, no shorter and certainly no longer. Speaking off the cuff – my strength – was not encouraged.

It went great, but I felt that had less to do with me than with the subject itself. First and last, it's relevant. People are engaged because what they're hearing is at once new to them yet so important to their overall health and well-being. I always explained enough science so it made sense, not so much that it bored or overwhelmed; you can get the essence without knowing what a cis polyunsaturated fatty acid is. It was my job – I believe it should always be the job of a physician and a patient advocate – to get people to understand what's likely to make them healthier or sicker, not just prescribe meds.

Within a day the video of the speech was posted on the TEDx YouTube site, and got some nice initial response, as did the videos of the seven other speeches that day.

Then, without warning, my talk began to take off. I don't know why. It had received zero coverage in the mainstream media. But the traffic was an order of magnitude more than anyone expected. Within a few days it grew to one hundred thousand views.

A quarter-million views.

A half-million views.

Holy cow! It was thrilling, regardless of the reason. I couldn't help but smile to think of Steve's ribbing when I exited the hotel elevator in Denver, and how I had better do a good job to get the expected – hoped-for! – fifty thousand views.

I thought of my dad, who had died in 2014 while the clinic was still in its early days. He always got excited about whatever my sister Jenna and I were doing. As the tally on my TEDx talk video continued to rise, Mom and I joked that if Dad were still alive, he would have been sitting at his computer, refreshing the screen over and over, watching the number of pageviews tick up and up and up. That would have become an obsession for at least a few days.

Not everyone who watched the video was a fan. A good deal of the traffic came from people who most definitely did *not* like my message: vegans. (Not all of them, of course, or even close to all.) In the comments, some among the most radical pro-vegans didn't bother to argue the science; there was none to argue. Their problem was that a low-carb diet tends to be animal-based, because the diet is nearly all protein and fat, and animals are nearly all protein and fat. So they resorted to personal attack. They called me vile names. They called me obese. That's right: I, a fit 130-pound woman, couldn't possibly know what I was talking about because I was . . . obese. Seriously? That was the best they could come up with? Weak as their counter was, it was spelled out in depressingly profane language. Brad and I forbid the kids from going to the page to see how I was being described.

Sometime later, a friend told me a piece of disturbing news. He had been in a meeting with two others – the president of a national grocery chain and a leader of the vegan community – and at one point the three of them watched a video, with doctored cuts of different talks I'd given so that I appeared obese. The president of the grocery chain commented on what an idiot I was. (He didn't know that one of the people he was talking to was a friend of mine.) It was ridiculous and sad, but I honestly didn't let it get to me personally;

136

it paled next to the kind of unfounded, empty-headed ridicule that my colleagues Steve Phinney, Gary Taubes, Nina Teicholz, and Jeff Volek, among other pioneers in the field of nutrition, had faced for years.

Most of the response to my talk was wildly positive.

The video hit a million views.

Two million.

It would reach close to eight million and counting.[32]

I was on a rocket ship.

As a doctor and a researcher, that was just about the last time I would take a deep breath for 18 months.

~

Based on their years of research and experience, Steve Phinney and Jeff Volek had a blueprint for how to educate patients on a low-carb lifestyle. They would teach the teachers (later, "health coaches") as the way to scale the message. It was called KetoThrive. At that point the use of technology to communicate with patients was in its infancy; the thought was that education by coaches would take place within healthcare facilities. Dr. Brittanie Volk, Jeff's former PhD student and a registered dietician, worked with them to help develop dietary, exercise, and behavioral change guidelines, which formed the basis of the app eventually used in our clinical trial.

Then Steve met Sami Inkinen, and that idea exploded into something much bigger.

---

[32] Editor's note: As of February 2024, the TEDx talk has over 11 million views.

Sami was a brilliant, energetic entrepreneur who had co-founded the online real estate site Trulia. Along with his business prowess, Sami was a triathlete who had won international competitions for his age group, and completed the legendary Hawaii Ironman competition seven times. He routinely worked out 12 hours a week. In the crucial final training days leading up to competitions, Sami followed the traditionally recommended route of "carbo-loading": eating bowls and bowls of oatmeal and pasta, loaves of bread, etc., ostensibly to maximize his energy stores. Sami had approximately 7% body fat, an impressively small amount.

In 2012, after Sami became a world champion triathlete, he was diagnosed with prediabetes. He had no family history of the disease.

What?

Sami ate well according to status quo guidelines . . . that were clearly wrong.

When Sami and his wife, Meredith Loring, planned a trip to Hawaii, they decided to forego flying for rowing, in a 22-footer. Sami and Meredith began training for an "open row," in the hope of breaking the mixed-couple world record for California-to-Hawaii. They were also inspired for other reasons: They wanted to raise awareness about the dangers of poor nutrition, particularly "the silent killer: sugar," and to show that you could exercise as much as 16+ hours per day without sugar. They were also inspired by Laura Hillenbrand's book *Unbroken: A World War II Story of Survival, Resilience, and Redemption*, about a very different trip in the Pacific.

They knew they would need to be in their best shape ever; for the many weeks of the row, their food intake would affect their muscle recovery and endurance.

Sami began investigating dietary impact, which led him to papers authored by Steve and Jeff. He read their book *The Art and Science of Low Carbohydrate Performance*. The more Sami read, the more he realized that the conventional wisdom about nutrition appeared to be not just misleading but flat-out wrong; that the typical carbohydrate-rich American diet was the problem. Sami tracked Steve down. They immediately connected, and Sami felt as if Steve could help – not only to get him and Meredith into their best shape but also to help Sami get out of his prediabetic state.

The more they talked, the more in sync they were, until Sami asked Steve to be his nutrition advisor for the row. Steve would advise Sami and Meredith on the optimal way to eat, for maximum performance and overall health. They discussed the micronutrients (e.g. sodium, magnesium) and food types (e.g. olive oil, nuts, beef) they would need, in which amounts. They tweaked the regimen, pre-row, to get the nutrition just right.

Following Steve's recommendations, Sami saw his body's production of insulin decrease as his blood sugar levels came down. Within weeks, he moved safely away from prediabetes. The competition, called Fat Chance Row, was his first major athletic competition on his new low-carb diet.

Sami felt *and* performed better than he ever had. He and Meredith arrived in Hawaii in 45 days, a world record for a two-person crossing.

Sami's eyes had been opened. He was lucky enough to have Steve to help him. But what about all the people with diabetes and prediabetes who lacked the resources and time to get help, let alone from Steve Phinney personally? Sami and Meredith started asking questions.

Why is the food supply so full of unhealthy and dangerous options?

Since healthy food is the main tool needed to diminish or reverse diabetes and decrease the need for diabetes medication, why isn't it more available?

Why aren't smarter, truer eating guidelines available? Especially when there are 400 million people worldwide with type 2 diabetes, and hundreds of millions more with prediabetes?

Sami – a natural-born innovator clearly not wired to accept the old "because that's the way it's always been done" explanation – had a new mission. He had personally experienced the reversal of a diagnosis that might have turned permanent, plus he had the impatience and resources to do something about it.

He wanted to reverse type 2 diabetes in millions of people.

Sami, Steve, and Jeff co-founded Virta, the company that was now going to provide the funding for our study. A for-profit startup, Virta was attempting to do what I had naïvely believed our not-for-profit healthcare system could: figure out ways to make people healthier, not just manage chronic illness. Their ambitious, explicitly stated goal for the company was to help reverse type 2 diabetes in 100 million people by the year 2025. At the heart of the strategy was a well-formulated ketogenic diet, but there had to be more to it than that. Virta would use technology – telemedicine, including monitors for blood sugar and other biomarkers, apps, and online communication – to help their patients achieve their goals. It was a classically Silicon Valley approach.

And there it was: the answer I'd been searching out.

Sarah, how do we make this scale?

With technology, that's how.

While there would very much be a human, in-person element to the study we were going to conduct, we aimed to translate as much of that as possible to the remote, online experience, maintaining the basic attentiveness and empathy that should be the essence of good medical care. What's the best way to monitor patients remotely? How could we bring needed information to them? How could we be the best possible care providers? We could talk to people about changing their diet but there was much more they needed to know as they moved to a low-carb lifestyle. How did they (and by extension, we, their supporters/advisors) deal with a lapse when they fell off their diet? How would we deal with patients going through life crises – divorce, death in the family, all the rest? We knew there was more to providing lasting care to patients than just focusing on food intake. It was a complex formula, all of it.

Before Steve and I had met in Denver, Virta was in preliminary talks to partner with various name-brand medical institutions – Harvard, Stanford, University of California at San Francisco, among others – but either the cost was too high, the commitment was too slow to develop, or the doubts and fears of their potential partners were signs of fatal status quo thinking. (*If this research is published, will it lead to my getting attacked? Will it upend my long-cultivated credibility? . . . yeah, no thanks.*) So Virta needed a partner – a "can do," scrappy partner, perhaps? – who could recruit patients and help run the trial. I was bursting to expand the scale of what I thought was possible. I was convinced it was possible. Here I stood, in Indiana, I hadn't gone to Harvard Medical School, I didn't have a name-brand platform, I had been periodically ignored, marginalized, or mocked by big places with household names. I was working to prove the science behind an idea that shouldn't have been a secret but often seemed so, a secret that could help millions – not just those at our clinic or within the greater Lafayette, Indiana region. I mean literally millions. And millions. Virta was the rocket ship to help with that goal.

Right before I met the Virta folks, they had been conducting a pilot program, partnering with a large healthcare system in the South. They had big dreams for their study; in reality, though, they got to treat only a few patients.

Brittanie – Britt – worked with a small group of patients, implementing nutritional changes, while also having very personal encounters with each patient. But at that point, it was a trial almost entirely free of any truly useful technology component. The hope was that the test could be expanded into a legitimate clinical trial that would include Virta's proprietary tech component.

The healthcare partner had over a million subscribers, and those in charge seemed legitimately eager to seek out the facts and the truth of what the trial was hoping to show. Virta wasn't going to be like a lot of Silicon Valley startups – "fake it till you make it" –

but needed to prove that their approach could work, at scale. They needed a study that was large enough and comprehensive enough to show that the protocols were safe and could be effectively implemented.

Unfortunately, because of personnel and logistical issues at the study venue, things turned frustrating fast. Britt and the patients were given no dedicated meeting room anywhere in this large healthcare system, so they had to use the waiting room in their clinic, and then only after hours. The tech component for Britt to communicate with patients was a rudimentary online spreadsheet that didn't work very effectively; email was another option, also not very personal. Then, when she wanted to implement the recommended diet for a segment of patients in the trial, the people in charge stonewalled her for months. The test fell apart.

Still, that's where Virta's first documented cases of diabetes reversal happened.

Fine, was my thought when I learned how Virta's attempts to work with big, scared, status quo-driven players had faltered and failed. *Those guys didn't want to be part of a groundbreaking way of addressing a generational health epidemic? Fine.*

So when I met Steve in Denver, either by accident or fate, I became the perfect Plan B – better than Plan A, I have to say – partly because of what I was interested in, partly because our clinic was already set up for what they had in mind.

Within a couple of weeks after first talking with Steve and being offered funding for a two-year trial, he and Britt flew to Indiana to meet with me. This was May 2015. Brad and I hosted them for dinner, and Tamara joined, too. Brad whipped up steak and his amazing grilled avocado with tapenade. Steve, a gourmet chef and lover of good food, had never before encountered grilled avocado; he fell in love – not with Brad, not with me . . . he loved that avocado!

Britt and I hit it off immediately. She was a PhD scientist and registered dietitian who was Virta's first official hire. She knew about me because Steve had encouraged her to watch my TEDx talk. She had left New Jersey, where her family lived, to run Virta's first big trial, the ultimately unsuccessful one in the South. And now, just months later, she was being asked, "Okay, can you move to Indiana?"

The morning after their arrival, Britt, Steve, and I spent time at the weight-loss clinic, and they met our whole great staff. Britt was psyched at how eager our clientele was to accept what the clinic was offering. And our staff was equally excited to meet the Virta people. At times my group and I had felt like lone pioneers, doing things that other physicians would have been scared to do, because the pushback would be so great.

Research on low-carbohydrate diets was also difficult in academia, where it was so hard (no, virtually impossible) to get grants to fund the work. Steve had encountered pushback throughout his career. By lunchtime, Jeff Volek and Jim McCarter, Virta's Head of Research, joined us and we were deep into discussing logistics – how we were going to get our protocol approved by the Institutional Review Board (IRB). An IRB is an oversight committee set up to ensure that all research done on humans is ethical and that patients have given informed consent. I was thrilled finally to meet Jeff in person; like me, he had a background in exercise physiology. It turned out that it was not our first meeting: a quarter-century earlier, while I was a grad student at Illinois State getting certified by the American College of Sports Medicine, my exam proctor was Jeff. It was strange and delightful for us to cross paths again. And there was the remarkable Jim McCarter, who grew up one town over from my hometown of DeKalb, Illinois, more strange and wonderful karma.

At one point, as we barreled toward a plan to get IRB approval, I had to interrupt.

"This is nuts!" I said. "Things like this just don't happen that fast."

Everyone there had done research, we all knew how long it took to get started – years and years, yet here we were talking about . . . months. Weeks?

By the time Britt got on the plane back to the South, she told me later, she knew she was moving to Indiana for the next year. It wasn't pleasant being away from family for so long, but she knew why she was doing it.

Once she relocated, we put her in a closet. That's not hyperbole – she was literally in a closet, windowless and tiny, because we didn't have extra space. But she was such a trouper. She and I felt a kinship because we each wanted to have an impact. Like me, she gave her all to everything. Like me, she hated to say no. Like me, she worked herself to the bone.

In addition to Britt, within weeks several people had moved to Indiana, including Dr. Amy McKenzie and Dr. Brent Creighton, who would be our first health coaches, followed quickly by Marcy Abner, Registered Dietitian (RD), Bobbie Glon (RN), and Theresa Link

(RD), all of whom had advanced training in metabolic health. The health coach has day-to-day interactions with patients through an app able to track biomarkers such as blood sugar, blood pressure, weight, and ketones. Patients are given the monitors they need to measure those markers, even an app-connected scale to track their weight.

Amy quickly became the experienced on-site eye on the trial. She was so passionate and I learned so much about research (remember, I was "just" a doctor before this). For the IRB, we had to write the whole protocol, describing everything we were going to do, and how. Steve took an apartment in town because he was visiting so frequently. We got deep into the details of designing the trial.

Even as I was getting to know Steve, I sometimes still pinched myself that *I was working with Steve Phinney*! One of the towering figures in the field, a man who had been fighting the fights that I was now fighting, only he'd been at it for decades.

~

Three months after that pivotal dinner in Denver with Steve and Tamara, we received IRB approval to begin the clinical trial I had dreamed about.

Yet our goal was unrealistic. More accurately, it was insane. Our biggest advantage, aside from experience with these issues and a great staff, was our waiting list. We had hundreds of names. But we wanted to enroll 500 participants. Could we do that in six months? Ridiculous. And my naivete was partly to blame.

When I first met Steve, I told him that our clinic had a waiting list of hundreds and hundreds of names, people desperate to get in. That was 100% true.

But it didn't mean that all those people would meet the inclusion criteria for our trial. We looked at health history. They had to have type 2 diabetes or prediabetes. Lots of people on the waiting list did not. They couldn't have had a cardiac event (a heart attack, for instance) in their recent past, or active cancer, or end-stage kidney disease. (We accepted people with other kidney issues, which are common among those with diabetes.)

We had a maximum age criterion of 65 years because the older people get, the likelier, obviously, they are to die. Age 18 was the youngest we would take; this wasn't a study of children. We did not include pregnant or lactating women because it was a population segment that would have required special monitoring and that had not been thoroughly studied for safety.

Even if an individual met all the criteria, it didn't mean that he or she could be convinced to take part in a trial scheduled to last two years, possibly more.

Some people on the list no doubt got frustrated that they had not gained admission to the clinic, and moved on. Some got calls from us and didn't call back.

The pool of eligible candidates was getting whittled down.

Jim McCarter stepped in and made crucial recommendations. We needed to invest money in radio ads and mailers, he said, and buy valuable mailing lists of people who ordered diabetes supplies. We needed to expand the audience of eligible candidates. We got the word out. Since we still had a clinic to run during all this, Virta hired someone to help our office staff to field all the new interests.

Over the course of eight months (mid-August 2015 to mid-April 2016), we did what seemed impossible: 465 people enrolled in the trial, for one site.[33] To our knowledge, there had never been a trial like it, with the potential to show just how well certain methods worked to help with weight loss and reversing diabetes. We had candidates from the St. Louis area, from Wisconsin, from Illinois. Of course the majority were from Indiana, from as far away as Indianapolis and beyond, all willing to make the drive. They wouldn't have to travel frequently to Lafayette – the idea, after all, was to provide information and support through technology-enabled remote care – but we would want to see them a couple of times a year.

As the trial start date approached, we were busy, excited, and underslept. Our staff was working their butts off but could barely handle the volume of inquiries. We had to find an Amazing Phone Person, and we did. Rachel Bolden was magic on the telephone. We were learning as we were going. We hired a certified diabetes educator with expertise in low-carb. We all got dedicated cell phones from Virta for calling patients and communicating with apps. We did practice runs, so we could simulate what it would feel like when we finally brought in patients. That was important for us and also for the patients: the ask of them was sufficiently great that we needed them to feel that we knew thoroughly what we were doing.

---

[33] We started enrolling patients in mid-August and got them going in the trial immediately, a "rolling start" as new patients began the program between August 2015 and April 2016.

When the trial started, it went like this: There was an experimental (or treatment) group and a control group. The experimental group was 378 strong, 262 who were diabetic and 116 who were prediabetic. They all received the same "treatment" of the very low-carb (ketogenic) diet and assigned health coaches.

Each participant was in daily contact with her or his coach. Each used monitors and apps. Each also had a choice of how to learn about the well-formulated ketogenic diet they were starting and how (and why) to incorporate it into their lifestyles. Some chose to come to the clinic for in-person instruction – the on-site cohort. Others chose to learn online by accessing our newly developed educational materials – the virtual cohort.

The control group consisted of 87 patients who all had diabetes. They were following the diet recommendations of the American Diabetes Association (ADA). We were not responsible for their care. They continued to meet with their own doctors and received standard diabetes education. They were given no app and no health coach with whom they would be in daily communication. We simply got their labs at the beginning of the study. We paid them to participate; essentially, to allow us to see the trajectory of their diabetes, weight, and other biomarkers. Their outcomes – how they did at the end of 10 weeks, and the end of Years 1 and 2 – were compared to the 262 members of the experimental group who had diabetes. The participants with prediabetes were analyzed separately.

This is how it worked. A patient in the on-site group – I'll call her Anne – would come to the clinic and I would do a brief history and physical and learn what medications she was on.

Anne would then meet in a group of about 20 patients for an in-person, two-hour session, led by a health coach, with me sitting in. On Mondays, groups started at 6:45 in the morning. We had thirteen groups per week.

A health coach was assigned to Anne; each coach was in charge of approximately 50 to 60 patients.

The initial carbohydrate goal for everyone was the same: try to get under 30 grams of carbs a day, with adjustments for individuals on vegetarian or vegan diets. The average daily American intake of carbohydrates is between 300 and 400 grams for men and 200 to 300 grams for women, so it was a huge shift. One can stay under 30 grams of carbs, for instance, with a cup each of zucchini and shredded cheddar cheese, ¾ cup of cauliflower rice, half an avocado, two cups of spinach, and two eggs. Meat, poultry, fish, bacon grease, butter, and olive oil all have no carbs.

Each person also had an individual protein goal linked to weight and gender.

Anne was given a starter kit – a cell phone-enabled scale and a monitor to check her levels of blood sugar and ketones (an elevated level indicates adherence to carbohydrate restriction). She would step on the scale and her weight automatically transferred to the app. We followed up by sending her educational videos and other content to watch or read, including my introductory lecture explaining the science and physiology behind what we were all engaged in.

As with every trial patient, Anne had to provide certain basic health information daily. She did not have to come to the clinic or see me to do it; with the finger stick we provided, she could do it via pinprick, at home.

If her blood sugar or ketone level on a particular day was unusual, I would know it and address her directly. For example, if Anne was on insulin and entered a morning blood sugar that was 20 points (20 mg/dL) lower than the previous day, I would adjust her insulin for that day. The app provided a way for us to communicate almost immediately and for me to adjust her medications safely and efficiently. She was in daily communication with her health coach, and occasionally with me, through the app. The initial contact was a one-on-one, get-to-know-you conversation between Anne and her coach. What do you do, when do you tend to eat, where do you eat, who's in your home this weekend – those sorts of things.

Anne's health coach was aware of the numbers, even though I was the one who could adjust medication. If Anne's blood sugar was low when she woke up in the morning, her coach could see that and contact her. "What did you do for dinner last night? I bet it went well." They could communicate about the experience. In this way, the monitoring of weight and health became less abstract and more personal, and certainly more personalized than it is in the once- or twice-a-year visit to the doctor's office. If Anne lost five pounds, wouldn't it be great to have both the data and a dedicated expert helping to figure out which behaviors of hers might have contributed to that? Within hours of eating, the metrics would register so that her coach was notified of some significant change, and could personalize the intervention. A dramatic increase in blood sugar . . . did Anne eat something new, or too much of something – nuts, for instance? (A common cause for someone trying to follow a very low-carbohydrate diet.) Her coach could advise alternatives, and Anne would feel a sense of control over the things that affected her physiology.

As needed, Anne and her coach communicated throughout the day via text message. Occasionally they would speak via phone or HIPAA-compliant video (privacy protected). As things progressed, the communication inevitably became more about troubleshooting and fine-tuning, though sometimes the messages could be rather urgent. It probably won't surprise you that a significant number of text communications to our coaches were initiated by patients as they were steering their cars into the drive-through of a fast-food chain. *Can I? Should I?*

The coach was there to provide daily guidance and encouragement. Anne might text, "Hey, can I eat turnips?" And her coach would reply (generally within minutes but sometimes up to a few hours) something like, "Yes, in moderation. Cooked turnips have four grams of carbohydrates per half a cup. Here are a couple of great turnip recipes." Or Anne would text, "I'm eating out at a new restaurant today," and her coach would walk with her through the menu choices.

The health coach became a friend to Anne, someone to rely on. All of us conducting the trial were sure that the coaches would be a key to our success. It was sad to think that this simple, obvious idea had been so lost in conventional healthcare that re-introducing it seemed practically radical. The rewards of this continuous care model are twofold: first and most importantly, patients live healthier and longer lives. Second, the healthcare savings are potentially huge – not only from the reduction or elimination of drugs for diabetes, but also the savings from other diseases that reverse, do not progress (or at least are less severe), or never happen in the first place, including diseases of the heart, liver, and kidney to name just a few that are so common in diabetic patients.

A lot of what we hoped to show in the trial was based, of course, in nutrition science. But we also wanted to show the importance of continuous human connection, either in-person or remote. Making a lifestyle change is hard. We couldn't just say, "Okay, here's what to do," and that's it, done. Even when we explained to patients the whys and hows, and provided them with clear instructions and options, we still had to be available to troubleshoot for them. Some individuals can, after education about the diet, maintain it without a lot of input from their healthcare providers. But many (most?) will require individualized continuous care, such as we used in our trial, with coaches and remote communication. And patients, including older patients, have embraced it. We were constantly working to improve and add to the healing and connecting aspects of healthcare.

Before the weekly group session, I would do a quick one-on-one with each of the 20 patients following this protocol, adjusting medications for those who needed it, and then they would proceed to their two-hour weekly meeting.

I loved being so involved, but for all that I was doing, my visits with the enrollees – seeing approximately 20 patients in a span of 40 minutes – reminded me of what I had so disliked about primary care: a lack of connection. So I sat in with the group I had just examined. It was in these gatherings that I got to know the patients, and they got to know me. The health coach led the conversation but I would chime in when appropriate.

That's generally how things went, week by week, for Anne and the other on-site enrollees.

The virtual cohort looked just like Anne's group except they did not come into the clinic for sessions. Their education, support, and medication adjustments were all done remotely – via the app and texting, with the same occasional call or video. They came to the clinic only for their physicals.

As part of our analysis, we compared the on-site and remote groups. That they were so similar both in their beginning characteristics and in their results gave us the confidence that we could scale our approach by using remote delivery.

~

To say the company was in its infancy is an understatement. Virta had a great idea, based on a book and lots of prior research. They had great people, with a similar goal and outlook. The app was being built and de-bugged as we were conducting the trial, as if we were driving a train on a track being laid down ten feet in front of us.

Still, the group meetings were delightful and intense, and even more engaging as patients came back week after week and we all got to know each other better. Within weeks of the first sessions, participants began seeing significant, sometimes profound reductions in medication. Each session became like a party. People were excited and energetic. Patient A

154

succeeded, then Patient D, then Patient K. It was more of the excitement from our obesity clinic, when we posted on the wall the pounds lost. For me, the fulfillment and joy never stopped, because I sat in on sessions with all 13 groups. I got to share in all the success. It was an honor. It was what I had *wanted* my medical career to be about. Many of the patients had taken to calling me Dr. Sarah, and I liked that. "Dr. Hallberg" felt too formal. I'm glad they respected me enough to say "Doctor" but I didn't want to be on a completely different level. This was a shared journey.

~

The hours were crazy. Endless. We were all working out of the IUH building. I'd see the "Virtans," as we took to calling them, all the time. We had rounds once a week, with the whole team – weight-loss clinic team and Virta health coaches – gathered in the doctors' lounge to discuss cases. It was a way for us all to learn what was or wasn't working with an individual, or across the board, and we used that information to build and improve the app. The session would last hours. We were all so overtaxed, the meetings were a mix of intensity and stupor, if that's possible. We would laugh at the compromised physical shape we were all in. If one person half-boasted, half-lamented, "I haven't slept in three days," the person next to him or her probably hadn't slept for four. Many of the health coaches were younger, having sacrificed a great deal to be there. Many had moved great distances from home – Connecticut, New Jersey, Ohio, Nebraska – for at least a year. They had left behind children, spouses, partners,

155

parents, other family members, friends, pets, homes, individual practices. One health coach who left behind her son and husband made teary phone calls home every chance she got. How hard was that? But they all believed in the mission and in doing right for the patients.

At this point, you might wonder: why did this treatment need to be so intense? Simple: many patients on diabetes medications need to have most of them removed or reduced in the first month or two when they start a ketogenic diet because this very low- carb diet and the medicines both lower blood sugar. If not done promptly, they'd be at risk for hypoglycemia: dangerously low blood sugar. If a patient broke the diet even briefly, blood sugar would go up and we'd have to add back some of those meds. In many patients, their meds needed changing multiple times per week. Steve Phinney liked to describe this as "outpatient intensive care." We were two doctors and six coaches managing almost 400 patients, seven days per week, but charting a whole new approach to type 2 diabetes.

And it was worth it.

One huge relief: no one from big industry or the big health associations was paying attention to us, at least not yet. At some point they would, because what we were doing would ultimately challenge so much of what they did and said; so much of their revenue could go up in smoke if people better understood the science of food, nutrition, dieting, carbohydrates, fat, and the rest. I knew how vicious some low-carb opponents had been with me and many of my colleagues.

Yet why would some of the smart people at places like the American Diabetes Association not examine or accept the notion of low-carb eating as a therapeutic option for people with diabetes? Given that mass-market farming practices and the commercialization of food products were in large part responsible for overloading the American diet with processed foods and carbohydrates, especially sugar, at the same time that obesity and diabetes exploded to epidemic proportions, why wouldn't they want to examine whether carbs might be seriously contributing to the problem?

There was evidence going back over a century that carbohydrate restriction worked. It was originally meant to help children with epilepsy, as well as to treat diabetes before we had insulin and other medication. But it began to show real promise for helping in other ways – not just for bringing down weight or controlling diabetes but improving other key health indicators, such as lowering risk factors for cardiovascular disease and helping certain nervous system disorders.[34]

We were trying to change the understanding of how things work, so that the general public would start avoiding the foods that were causing so much harm and demand foods more beneficial to their long-term health,

---

[34] The case for various carbohydrate-restricted diets goes back to at least the mid-1800s when a British undertaker named William Banting became one of the first known people to popularize a low-starch diet. At his doctor's advice, Banting cut out bread and beer, also sugar and potatoes, and witnessed tremendous results. He felt better and within a year had lost 35 pounds. This is a fun and interesting story about Banting: Jones, PA. "William Banting, Early Champion of the Low-Carb Diet." *Mental Floss.* August 2, 2016. mentalfloss.com/article/83944/william-banting-early-champion-low-carb-diet

at which point industry would accommodate, as they do. There were so many big implications to what we were doing: for individual health, for population health, for the exploding cost of healthcare, for the environment, for farming practices. It would impact so many companies and multiple industries.

The ADA had good reasons to take its time in acknowledging what our team and I – and so many others – were doing. Of course it did. Where does the ADA get its money? For one, the pharmaceutical industry. And if people are reversing their type 2 diabetes through a whole-food diet and don't need their insulin and diabetes meds anymore, that removes a major revenue source.

Over time, as the health coaches and I grew more comfortable around each other, I realized how real I could be with them. We all enjoyed people but sometimes one of us just didn't want to deal, and the others would take over. Yet even if I was feeling stressed or pissed, I tried never to let it affect how I was with patients. No matter what preceded it, right before I entered a group session, knowing who was on the other side of the door and what had brought them there, I would always take a deep breath, re-set, and enter saying, "Good morning, everybody!" Nothing was going to get in the way of their belief in my belief in them.

~   ~   ~

Chapter 15

Exhaustion, Recognition, Almost

Perfection

When done right, there's a lot of happiness in diabetes and obesity care. We got to experience a lot of joy.

We were seeing many signs of success, often amazing success, with the trial treatment patients while the trial control group (those who were "just" being seen in clinic and by the diabetes dietitians) remained stable, at best. The former group had the advantage of day-to-day communication with their health coaches who knew about their situation and had incentive to care about it. They had that biomarker feedback loop, available to them all the time. And, of course, they were getting the right nutrition guidance – carbohydrate restriction – for their disease.

One woman, 60 years old and close to 300 pounds, had started in the treatment group in a scooter chair. In the previous few years, she had deteriorated from being able to walk, to needing a cane, to needing a walker, to needing a motorized chair. Within three months of joining our trial, she gave up the chair and walked again, without a walker or cane – a huge shift in mobility, independence, and enthusiasm for life. We all celebrated with her.

We had two people each born with one kidney, and each had suffered some kidney failure because the remaining one was overly taxed. Ten weeks after starting the trial with us, the labs for both of them registered normal kidney function.

Everyone gets excited when they lose weight, of course. But in the group sessions, or sometimes on check-in phone calls, we had NSV – "non-scale victories" – because not all triumphs register on the scale.

I'm all the way off insulin. My blood sugars are normal now.

I went to the beach with my family and I got up out of the sand by myself.

I bought these pants in a regular store.

I saw my penis for the first time in forever.

I took my first flight where I didn't have to ask for a seatbelt extender.

I was able to go on a rollercoaster with my son and I could see how much it meant to him.

This is the way my grandmother used to cook.

These were moments to be celebrated, worthy of joyful tears, by the individuals and all of us who were there to support them. Lots of the motivation and ultimate gratitude came from the patient's child or spouse/partner. The husband or wife of a patient would come in and tell us, "You saved our lives. I was losing him/her." Or "I thought my wife/husband would die within a year, and now I have her/him back." One patient was about to sell his beloved motorcycle because he had gained so much weight that he couldn't ride anymore. I was there when he announced that he had lost enough weight to take up riding again. Another man had tears in his eyes when he went off insulin and told us his doctor had once told him that his diabetes would get progressively worse and he would never be able to stop using insulin.

Stories like these were happening every day. The power of these triumphs offset the exhaustion we all felt daily.

~

Part of the success was from our emphasis on patient choice. A one-size-fits-all approach would not work. Different things worked for different people. Some patients needed to start off with modifications to our low-carb guidelines because of "problems" they felt came along with a truly low-carb diet. It wasn't necessarily the diet itself, but often social or family issues. For example, some patients felt embarrassed or weird ordering a low-carb meal at a restaurant because if they then asked for butter, they felt they would be fat-shamed because they were already overweight. So much empathy was required on our part, and at times I found myself taking their pain home with me. How could we improve what we were doing? The key was always in talking with patients, genuinely understanding them, then educating them. They deserved to know the choices that were right for them.

Amy and I went shopping at every single grocery store in Lafayette, to understand the options and prices. The patients in the clinic ranged from those who had the money to pay for more expensive food to those on Medicaid. An important part of our personalized care was understanding each patient's food budget, then working with them based on that. We alerted some patients about the gigantic $1 bags of frozen vegetables at Walmart, which was profoundly helpful to them. At times we would help them create a menu. I developed a relationship with the owners of one grocery store and they kindly allowed us to label approved foods for our patients to purchase. In time, many of the local restaurants started offering low-carb options. At one place it was crustless pizza. At another it was zucchini noodles, or the entree on a bed of spinach instead of rice. In an exciting grassroots way, the status quo was changing, at least when it came to menu options in the eating establishments in Lafayette, Indiana.

Skepticism about what we were doing in the trial was always there, just outside our walls. But the fact that there were people on the outside willing to help and who did help – that was inspiring. And necessary. Most importantly, the unbelievable hard work that our patients were doing to adjust their diets and lives: that was the most inspiring of all.

~

In May 2016 the ADA included bariatric surgery in its standard of care treatment for diabetes – a good thing because it meant a backing off from the approach that diabetes was a progressive disease and all you could hope to do was manage it. But they still did not include a low-carb diet. Were they serious? They endorsed major, very expensive surgery ahead of a doable, sensible dietary change?

For me, that was the last straw.

Big Diabetes could ignore the expanding

evidence on low-carb for diabetes therapy, but I wasn't going to ignore them. I co-wrote an op-ed, with Dr. Osama Hamdy, medical director of the Obesity Clinic Program and Inpatient Diabetes Program at the Joslin Diabetes Center at Harvard Medical School, published in *The New York Times*. The title was simple and to the point, "Before You Spend $26,000 on Weight-Loss Surgery, Do This." [35]

I was pleased with the exposure we got in *The New York Times*, but I should have known that institutional thinking wasn't giving up without a nasty fight. The *Times* piece documented how our clinical trials and others, including studies from decades before, had persuasively shown the efficacy of the low-carb diet to undo the damaging effects of diabetes – and yet the remarkable benefits of those studies were questioned, demeaned, or ignored in favor of the low-fat diet, which had been shown just as persuasively to have almost *no* chance of helping those in need. Wait – was the *Times* really joining the fight against status quo, wrongheaded thinking? Um . . . not exactly. They let a columnist, the notoriously anti-low-carb Gina Kolata, write a follow-up hit piece. Such a response was unusual to begin with – a full-length article "rebuttal" rather than just, say, a letter or shorter piece; never mind the cherry-picked data she used to diminish the benefits and viability of a low-carb diet. Kolata's

---

[35] "Before You Spend $26,000 on Weight-Loss Surgery, Do This." *New York Times*, September 10, 2016. nytimes.com/2016/09/11/opinion/sunday/before-you-spend-26000-on-weight-loss-surgery-do-this.html.

agenda (or agendas) was apparent when she referred to my friend Osama Hamdy, a man, as "a medical director at a major medical institution" (Harvard), while calling me – *the lead author* of the paper in question – "an osteopath from Indiana."

Where do I start? Is that sexist? Elitist? I had the exact same job (leader of an obesity/diabetes program) as my esteemed colleague Dr. Hamdy, and I too was at an esteemed institution – Indiana University Health.

Unreal.

~

As our clinical trial progressed, some day-to-day responsibilities slowed a bit for me. Groups met less frequently. I no longer had to do the history and physical for patients because everybody was already enrolled.

Still, the trial, combined with other work at the clinic, was consuming, often ridiculously non-stop. I woke up at 4:30 every morning, knowing I would be going for 15+ hours of work that day, not counting my responsibilities to my family, and my desire just to be with them. I tried going to the occasional barre class but it was tough to find time, and tough to let go when I did. My own physical well-being was not high on my list of priorities. That kind of ignoring of self was exactly what we advised our patients *not* to do themselves. It was all enough to make me question what I had gotten into.

What kept me sane was the mission.

I'd get to the clinic and see a patient smiling and know it was related to something that our team had helped her or him with. That's all it took for me to flip the switch for the day, knowing I was doing the right thing.

And I needed to remind myself of all that, each and every day, because the fatigue was building. One day, our busiest to that point, with more patients coming and going than we'd ever seen, I began to lose it. By late afternoon I was overwhelmed, burnt to the core. I walked past Britt's windowless closet and opened the door. I saw her, far from her family, looking up at me; Steve Phinney, in town that week and also far from his family, sat beside her in the tiny space, also looking up at me.

I wasn't sure if I was seeing their exhaustion, or my own reflected back to me in their faces.

"I don't know if I can do this anymore," I whispered, on the verge of tears. "I can't keep this pace up. It's overwhelming."

I will never forget the look on their faces. They didn't launch into a *Just-a-little-bit-more-Sarah!* pep talk. No *Come-on-you're-awesome!-you-can-do-it!* That was the last thing I needed to hear then. I needed just to hear someone feel bad for me because I was truly overwhelmed. A lot like how patients need their doctors just to hear what it is they're facing.

Not surprisingly, that's exactly what I got from Britt and Steve. They both wore the same beautiful expression of utter sympathy and empathy. I could see in their eyes complete understanding of where I was at that exact moment, because it's pretty much where they were, too.

Britt nodded. Steve nodded.

"Okay, we're going to change this," said Steve. "We've got to find you help for what you need."

But that *was* precisely what I needed – just that. An appreciation by others of what I was going through. As long as I had that, as long as I had seen that in their eyes immediately and authentically, I could keep on going.

Another crazy day, but I knew I could handle it.

~

I attended barre class more regularly, but with so much work always waiting, I never stayed the whole hour. I would leave class after 45 minutes, thoughts gnawing at me that the next 15 minutes were better spent at the clinic serving others, not here getting my own body and head straight.

But relief was coming. The trial had a defined end date, the spring of 2018._[36] In the meantime, I would do everything I could to spend every possible moment with my family. I felt I had really short-changed them since the trial started.

As for time truly for myself: that seemed an almost laughable concept. My one indulgence was shopping at Goodwill. I'm a big believer in the idea that just because you can doesn't mean you should. I could buy nice *new* clothes – but did I really need to? I took great pleasure in stocking up my wardrobe with items from Goodwill. Shopping there was *my* time, my mental relief. I became a Goodwill addict. I found it therapeutic to go through the racks and bring home ten pieces of new clothing, all for a grand total of $30. Soon enough, practically every piece of clothing I wore to work came

---

[36] The study was later extended to spring 2021, for a total of five years.

166

from Goodwill. I happily boasted to my patients that I shopped at Goodwill. Then, when I'd bump into one of them there, she would come up to me and say some version of the same thing, "Dr. Sarah! I didn't think you were telling the truth!"

"Of course I was," I told them.

~

As I was getting more known, from speeches and conferences and the TEDx talk, I did the opposite of what you're supposed to: I withdrew. I was never big on social media but now the more public my profile, the less I wanted it. I feared that if I did use social media more, my big public personality would take over, and Sarah Hallberg would become more about the social media person and presence, less about the science.

Once, I gave a talk at the American Heart Association in Chicago, where my daughter Ava, age 13, had joined me. Afterward, on the way home she and I went to Costco, and while we were shopping for macadamia nuts, a man approached me.

"Oh, my god," he said. "Are you Dr. Hallberg?"

"Yes," I said, warily. I was slightly panicked, wondering where I might know him from. He didn't look familiar. Was he a hater?

"My wife and I just got done watching one of your videos," he said. "We're huge fans. You've changed my wife's life."

Ava stood there with her mouth open.

"Oh, my gosh," I said, relieved as much as gratified. "Well, thank you for saying that!"

When the man left, Ava looked at me and said,

"Oh, my god."

That was nice.

But there were always more fights to fight. The status quo doesn't go quietly.

I was invited to testify before a Congressional working group about nutrition. Then I got disinvited, for reasons I can only speculate. Then I was re-invited.

It wasn't the first time my visibility and experience irked or troubled status quo thinkers in the fields of nutrition, weight loss, obesity, and diabetes. There were multiple occasions where I was asked to write an article, or submit a paper, and was promised placement or told excitedly about the fast-tracking of it . . . only to learn, without valid explanation, that it was canceled or postponed indefinitely or "not right for us" or ignored, especially disheartening developments when the information had the power to help people *now*. So many food industry people – either academics funded by the industry or scientists expressly employed in the industry – are reputed to be sound nutrition scientists but are clearly indebted to those who pay them. In a word, they're shills. A journalist interviewed me extensively for an article on low-carb, for a magazine in the food industry. I was excited to think that they were going to give it serious coverage.

I hadn't learned my lesson about not getting my hopes up too high or too early.

I believed the magazine piece was coming out soon. When it didn't, I emailed the journalist. She wrote back that she had had some "unusual" pushback from the editors, and would have to interview me some more. Fine.

When several more months passed with no word, I emailed the journalist again.

She wrote back, distraught. They did not want my interview in the article. The journalist said that the editor confessed that it wasn't the low-carb point of view they were trying to remove. It was me. Dr. Sarah Hallberg.

Apparently, they didn't like my "bad mouthing" the Guidelines – in the TEDx talk and then *The New York Times* op-ed, I would guess.

They wanted someone else interviewed in my place. The journalist, deeply concerned about the ethical connotations of scrubbing an expert that the editor had originally agreed was okay, quit the assignment. I was so impressed with her for keeping her moral compass in check when doing so came with real sacrifice.

I wrote back to the journalist, thanking her for sharing her fiasco. It was incredible, and sad, and unsurprising. "There's a lot of money at play here," I wrote to her, "and when the powers that be have been giving bad advice (they absolutely have), then there will be a lot of heads to roll. I just can't believe the lengths they will go to suppress a) help for the patients they are supposed to be advocating for and b) science."

I'd had the gall to point out that what those powers had been saying for decades, and were still saying, was inconsistent with the best science available.

Here's the best one: one of the officers of the ADA, I learned, had portrayed me to his colleagues as a lunatic who no one should ever work with.

The fight continued.

~

When our clinical trial first started, my longtime IUH colleagues kept saying, "Oh, you're going to leave and work for Virta."

I was a little hurt by their assumption but really more startled by it. "No way!" I told them. "I am *not* leaving." The weight-loss clinic was my baby, and I was confident I could do both.

Eventually, though, as I saw what we were achieving with technology, the success we were having while still maintaining a very personal, often daily connection to patients, I grew increasingly frustrated by what we *weren't* doing at IUH. For example, I saw that a patient in the obesity clinic (not in the trial) who I thought was on her way to improvement had not come around for many months. I wanted to know how she was faring. Had she enjoyed success? Had she failed? How was she defining success or failure?

Yes, I could try to call her. But that's not how traditional medicine is set up to work. Technology was the way, the only way, that this kind of healthcare – maybe most healthcare – would scale.

There seemed no end in sight on the work, my obligations to both the IUH clinic and Virta. I plugged along like this for months until I had to admit that enough really was enough. Something had to give.

Sami and Steve flew in from California. Jim came in, too. They said to me almost the exact version of what Steve and Britt's expressions had once said to me. *We feel you. We hear you.*

The actual words? "Tell us what your dream job is," said Sami, "and we'll make it happen."

Oh, my god, was he serious?

Talk about feeling appreciated! I knew enough about Sami by then to know that, yeah, he was absolutely serious. So were Steve and Jim. In the short time the company had been in business, they had developed a culture that practiced what it preached. It wouldn't work if they were kind to their clientele – patients – yet not to those people delivering compassionate healthcare. I knew that when employees had a crisis with their kids or their own health, Virta's response was not, *Oh god, you can't do this now, we're a startup!* It was, *You're valuable to us. How can we support you?*

Hearing someone say, "Tell us what your dream job is and we'll make it happen" – not just imagining someone saying that – isn't that everyone's fantasy?

I was offered a contract to be a Virta employee, based right there at IUH.

It was the technology that convinced me to say yes. By this point I had had enough experience in healthcare to understand the limitations of brick-and-mortar in offering patient support; I had had enough exposure to the financial limitations of trying to do extensive one-on-one visits with everyone. No matter your good intentions, you simply can't "touch" everyone you need to every single day. True, not everyone needs that touch. But my experience had taught me that many, if not most, do, and the cohort I was dealing with did maybe more than most. The ones who need that regular touch and get it are the ones who so often show palpable success.

Technology was the best available way to overcome those limitations.

I couldn't completely leave IUH because I had a deep attachment to the weight-loss clinic. Virta appreciated that, and allowed me to stay part-time, while also being a Virta employee. Initially I was in charge of setting up protocols for patient care, but then Virta hired an amazing endocrinologist who assumed that responsibility. I helped out with sales and marketing, when needed. I got on sales calls to field clinical questions about our trial from physicians, nurses, dietitians, pharmacists, and the like. I did on-site events and webinars. Through Virta, I got the opportunity to travel extensively – often to San Francisco, where they were headquartered at the time, but also to other cities around the country. I spoke at conferences or smaller gatherings of physician groups. I spoke at many medical school grand rounds. I was engaged in our research but also asked to do lots of outreach, talking about the science of nutrition, healthy eating, insulin, obesity, diabetes. I loved reviewing the science with doctors who were eager to learn more, and I loved – though this may sound surprising – when my professional colleagues in the audience pushed back at me. It meant they were really listening, that there was some entrenched idea that needed to be dislodged. I was there to show them, in detail and with solid scientific evidence, what was sound about our approach and so unsound about previous conventional nutritional "wisdom."

While presenting at one dinner, I had thought the doctors seated around the room, all of whom worked in obesity medicine, would be naturally friendly to the concepts I was presenting. But at one point I got into a disagreement with a member of the audience – I don't remember now what it was. I offered multiple pieces of scientific evidence to support what I said; he responded mostly with emotion.

As he continued, two of my Virtan colleagues rose from their seats and began talking over the man, trying to shield me from conflict.

"It's okay," I told them calmly, gesturing for them to sit. "Don't worry. I've got it."

I appreciated their concern – not wanting me to be upset (I wasn't) or feel picked on (I was used to it). They didn't know me well enough yet to realize how much I relished being in that very spot.

Because I loved research and I was the principal investigator of our big trial, I also couldn't help coming up with new ideas. I was always telling people, "This is a question we need to ask" or "This is a project we need to do." To their credit, Virta encouraged me to keep pushing. We did a review of the ADA guidelines and diabetes reversal. I joined in on research looking at patients with type 1 diabetes eating low-carb.

As much as I was still working, some of the load had been lightened. Despite more traveling, I was able to spend more time with Brad and the kids. I was doing what I loved and felt as if I were helping lots of people, and working on methods that could help a substantially greater number.

And then, almost impossibly, things got even better: I found out that I had been awarded an Aspen Health Innovators Fellowship. My colleague Jim McCarter had kindly nominated me many months before. It meant I would meet annually for five years and work with other young(ish) health professionals on projects and ideas to improve, even revolutionize, healthcare in the US.

It was another dream come true.

If that wasn't enough – and it was, all of it was – I received an email from a recruiter inquiring if I was interested in an executive position at one of the famous tech companies.

It was a great time of life. It felt almost like a dream.

~   ~   ~

PART 3

CHANGE MYSELF

After a while, just staying alive becomes a full-time job.

- Michael Zadoorian

Chapter 16

Before and After

This is the way Brad and I "preferred" to die:

We're both 95 years old. We're driving back home following an amazing week of skiing. We get into a fiery car crash. No funeral necessary, no bodies for the kids and grandkids to deal with. Close enough to home that they don't have to go far to view the last moment. Brad and I don't have to watch each other slowly die.

The perfect way to go. It was a running joke between Brad and me.

I was not obsessed with death, though a doctor encounters so much more of it than the average person. Whenever our kids would freak out about death, the way kids do – *Oh god, what if something happens to you?* – yearning for comfort from Brad or me, I was ready: "You guys don't have to worry. That's why your mom and dad take such good care of themselves. You have the healthiest mom in the world. The only parent who's healthier is Dad, *maybe*. But that's it."

~

June 30, 2017. I was pumped for a great day.

The morning sun was intense, matching my mood as I sat in my car in the parking lot of the clinic, pausing for a moment to take a deep, satisfied breath. I had just presented before the Independent Review Board, advocating for an extension of our clinical trial, from two years to five, and it had gone well. If I'm being honest? It went incredibly well. I rocked the presentation. So I was relieved about that, and especially excited about what lay just ahead: the long July 4th weekend, which meant our annual party (then in its seventh year) *and* Brad's and my 20th wedding anniversary. Through kids and work, changing jobs and schools, moving from city to city early in my medical career, family illness and death, along with other family dramas, Brad and I had been through a lot, as of course have so many married couples, but we always found our way back to each other. *For better, for worse, for richer, for poorer, in sickness and in health.* Reaching the milestone of twenty years was something to celebrate.

I rewarded myself with a mid-morning exercise class. During planks I felt an ache in my upper chest, something I'd vaguely noticed for the last few weeks, but it was bearable, probably due to my increased workout regimen. I was the healthiest person I knew (except possibly for Brad) and pushing myself physically was part of who I was.

I stopped back at the office. I mentioned to Tamara the tech company recruiter calling me about an executive job.

"What?" she said, part excited, part nervous. "What will you do?"

"Are you kidding? My life is great. I would never consider changing course. What could get better?"

My response is burned into my mind. It's shocking to remember how I once felt about my life. The memory comforts me and tortures me.

~

At around 2:00 in the afternoon, from the basement of our home, I phoned a Virta colleague, for our twice-a-month call to discuss trial patients. The call turned strange almost immediately. I don't say that from memory. I was told it much later. I myself have only a fragmented recollection of the next twenty-four hours and beyond. What's there is in spurts, or as if in a fog, but no, not really. Most of what I write about the days that followed that phone call is courtesy of others.

I started to talk and right away thought it sounded odd. I recall thinking – or I *think* I recall thinking – *Oh, my god, he'll think I'm drunk.* I felt as if I were slurring my words, not making sense. I thought I kept saying, "Okay, wait a minute. Let me start over." I continued babbling. I remember looking at the phone. At some point I got so freaked out, I hung up on him.

No one knows how much time passed until Noah, my oldest at 14, found me in the basement. Apparently I started yelling incoherently. I have no recollection.

The next thing I remember:

Highway. Car. Brad and me. I have a flash of that moment, like a snapshot, slightly blurry but real. Brad is saying, "I don't think we can take you to urgent care." Something like that. I don't trust my memory of what he said. Again, Brad: "We're taking you to the emergency room."

That's it for memories in the car.

The next thing I recall is the trauma bay at the hospital, IUH Arnett. I don't remember our pulling up. Or getting out of the car. I was babbling, that much I knew. Brad says I kept saying something over and over again but it was incomprehensible. I am fascinated to know where my mind went in that terrified and unchecked moment.

The strangeness I felt in the trauma bay hit a whole other level because I had taken care of patients there. IUH Arnett was our primary affiliated hospital, though in recent years I had spent little time there as I reduced my hospital presence to almost nothing and saw patients only in the clinic. In fact, one of the last times I set foot inside the ER was not as a doctor but as the mother of a patient. At 3½ years old, Luna fell and hit her head while playing with Ava and suffered a grand mal seizure. When Brad called me at work to tell me, he started with, "Sarah, you need to sit down. Luna is here with me but she is not conscious. We're in the ambulance on our way to the ER." I sped to the hospital, another car ride I can barely remember. Luna remained unconscious for more than an hour, only starting to come around while she was in the CT scanner. I've never been so happy to see a CT scan procedure ruined. She had suffered a serious concussion. Thankfully, there seem to be no lingering effects.

Now, four years after that awful day, I was back in the trauma bay, a place layered with that extra dread for me. Brad was with me. He was calling and texting those who needed to know – Mom, first and foremost.

I know from Mom that she assumed, or wanted to assume, that it was just a really nasty migraine. She was rehearsing in her head the speech she planned to give me about overworking. Later, Brad called Mom to say they were going to do a scan and an MRI.

As I was taken to get an MRI of my head, Brad had to make a fast decision. He was told that my symptoms were almost certainly caused by a stroke. They told him that if there was no bleeding in my brain, then he had to decide if he wanted me to get "clot-busting" medication, which could save my life – but which also came with a 10% chance of worsening disability or death. Poor Brad. *For better, for worse, in sickness and in health.* As a non-medical person, his first reaction was to call my sister Jenna, a nurse practitioner in San Francisco. His second reaction was to call Tamara, my close friend and colleague, the person with whom just hours before I had shared my joy at my perfect life.

I don't know what decision Brad ultimately landed on; I presume he told them they could give me the medication.

But then it didn't matter. Once they had the result of the MRI of the brain and CT scan of the lungs, they could see that things were far worse than a stroke: a large brain tumor that caused the swelling, as well as a smaller brain tumor. Plus, a primary lung tumor and so many more as well.

Brad called Mom again to say there was something on my brain. He was crying by this point, and Mom, wrapping herself in understandable denial, still couldn't believe it was anything awful. It couldn't be. It made no sense.

A flurry of activity.

Brad staring off, deer-in-the-headlights look.

An IUH administrator appeared. *Why is he here?* I'm guessing I thought.

Brain tumor.

Emergency surgery.
What? How terrible! Who?

As a massive dose of steroids started to work, decreasing the swelling around the large tumor taking up residence in my brain, I eventually realized they were talking about me.

They believed I had lung cancer, and the tumors in the brain were the result of the lung cancer metastasizing. They didn't know it for sure because they had yet to get back the pathology report. With the CT scan of the chest and the MRI of the head, they could guess. Usually you don't get brain cancer metastasizing to the chest. And if you have metastatic lung cancer, the first place it often spreads is to the brain. Lung to brain, not brain to lung. Since my chest was full of tumors, that was the logical conclusion.

No, I never smoked.

The next thing I remember was arguing with my husband.

"They're wrong," I kept telling Brad. "They're wrong!"

A computer monitor sat on the nearby rotating desk, with my chart onscreen. "Swing that over for me," I told him. He didn't want to. I can't blame him now for refusing. But right then I was angry. It was just the two of us in the room.

"Brad, bring the computer over here," I snapped. "I want to look at it myself!"

After more hesitation and weakening counterarguments, Brad reluctantly swung the computer toward me. I looked at the images and data and words on screen. I had been in this ER room many times before, this was my hospital, I was a physician.

Only now I was a patient.

"This is a mistake!" I yelled at Brad. "This is all a big mistake! This is not happening. I'm healthy!"

I know from Tamara, who came to the hospital as soon as Brad called and was with me during most of my stay, that I was trying to figure things out, to solve the problem before us. I had a seizure – why? Tamara says I was pushy and forceful and demanding, the way I can often be in more mundane moments, but now I was borderline out of control.

Could it be something other than cancer, like a fungal infection? Was that possible? What other outcome could I hope for?

~

The surgeon entered. I didn't know him, though I knew so many of the surgeons and other doctors at Arnett.

"We're going to operate in the morning on that big mass," he said, in the clipped, I-just-told-you-all-you-need-to-know way of surgeons.

They had concluded that the larger of the brain tumors – posterior, left – was too big to shrink with steroids alone. They weren't concerned at the moment about the smaller one. If we didn't get the big one out right away, I'm told the doctor warned, "that's it."

That's it.

Would I have ever used that wording with a patient or their loved ones?

Brain surgery was scheduled for the morning.

I continued my belligerence. I know they drugged me, pain medicine along with steroids. I don't remember anything at all about that night or being in the ICU.

What was it like to be my husband that final day in June, the day before my brain surgery, a day that started out so perfect and turned so dreadful?

I can only imagine what that night with me in the ICU was like for dear Brad. His healthy, seemingly unstoppable wife of almost twenty years was scheduled for brain surgery. My sister had arrived by now; she had jumped on the first flight from California. Mom was home with the kids, though I shudder to imagine how she distracted herself and them, given the situation. I can't even fathom it. I don't want to. All of our close friends showed up to support Brad that night, and for that I am forever grateful. I was told that a lot of the forced conversation revolved around my sister's very trendy new shoes.

~

The following morning I was wheeled toward the operating room. This I kind of recall. Brad was beside me. I said something or attempted to say something about credit cards – that I wanted a friend to take my credit card and go shopping with Ava. An off-the-wall comment under the circumstances, but I'm guessing I understood the gravity of the situation and my focus was on comforting my daughter, a teenager. Shopping makes everything better, doesn't it?

As I was being taken into surgery, I already knew something about lung cancer diagnoses: most people are dead within a year. For the very lucky ones, it's usually just a few years. I knew what treatments for hopeless situations were like. I'd seen this scenario too many times. Dealing with patients and talking to family members who were really suffering, as they watched their terribly sick family member suffer. I didn't want any of that for myself. I had always vowed – granted, it was abstract then – that I would never do that to my family, or to me. It wasn't the horrible things that were going to happen to me that I dreaded, but the horrible things my kids would have to watch.

In the OR, I recognized the neurosurgeon from the day before. The anesthesiologist was unfamiliar to me. I knew so many surgeons and anesthesiologists, how was it that I had gotten two strangers?

Before I went under, I remember – this I vividly remember – instructing the anesthesiologist, "Don't let me die. I'm a mom."

~

The first memory I have, post-brain surgery, is of me screaming.

I woke up exhibiting no neurological issues. None. No weakness, no slurred speech other than from the drugs. No other symptoms. I guess I had luck on my side – that, and a good surgeon.

I remember Tamara in the room, and an IUH administrator. So many people, their presence all telling me what I already knew, but also had not fully absorbed.

I remember someone saying how lucky I was because if this had all happened ten years earlier, I'd be dead already. That was a perfect example of how things can and do change in medicine. How they can move forward *when the status quo is not working*.

But of course they merely meant surviving the first twenty-four hours. Still, something to be grateful for. Over the next 48 hours, the medical team ran through neurological tests. They would wake me every couple of hours and run a whole neurological exam – flashing light in my eyes, turning my head to follow it, telling me to keep my eyes shut and stick out my tongue, having me move each limb. I'd administered the same tests myself on countless patients.

I was on high-dose steroids, high-dose pain medication, anti-seizure meds. I'm sure the combination was a big reason I was sleeping the whole time and have so little memory of the aftermath.

I remember looking at my fingernails and thinking, *I have the best nails in this hospital. How can I be sick? I'm sure they never see someone with nails like mine.*

~

Could it be something else? Was there even a little chance? I was desperate for the answer to be yes. Not only because, as a doctor, I was always questioning the status quo but because, well, *everyone* in my position wants an answer different from the one they're getting. Of course we do! Donald, the patient I wrote about at the very start of this book, the one I waited to speak to myself and try to console even though I was in labor with Luna: he wanted a very different answer from the one I had to give him.

There were so many spots on my lung and brain, it looked as if it *could* be a fungal infection called cryptococcus. A couple months before, over spring break, Brad and the kids and I had vacationed in the Utah desert, an environment where you might get such an infection. I pushed the radiologist. And pushed.

"It's possible," he relented. He looked unconvinced.

Later I asked the oncologist. "Could it be cryptococcus?"

"It's so unlikely," he said, almost apologetically. His name was Ti Jones (still is). He's a good doctor and a good person. I understood the position he was in.

Still.

"Just tell me there's a *chance*," I said.

He looked at me. "Okay," he said. "There's a chance."

I told him I refused to do chemo. If my logic seems muddled, you're right.

"Okay," he said.

That evening, I studied my chart on my laptop, researching more. If it was the cancer they suspected, I had a five percent chance of living five years.

The physician in me took over. The realist. This was really happening.

~

On the Fourth of July they were going to discharge me from the hospital.

We still didn't have the pathology report back to confirm what they thought I had.

I dressed to leave. I was anxious to go but – as I knew only too well – there would be the usual delay in the discharge processing. I may have been shocked, panicked, drugged, but I could not countenance wasting time. Anticipating my reaction to any delay, Brad nervously approached. "Sarah, don't throw a fit," he implored. "These people have taken really good care of you. Please don't throw a fit." I was in no mood to listen to the advice, never mind that it was sound, never mind that it was my devoted husband who always had my best interest in mind.

"No, I'm done!" I said. "I'm ready to go! I'm not staying here! I don't have much time left so I'm not staying here one more second!" Which of course stressed Brad even more. I went from yelling at him to yelling at the nurses to just yelling in general.

I don't know who was happier about my leaving – me or the staff.

For our annual Fourth of July party, our friends and their families come over, play games, we make and eat great food and drink champagne, and top the celebration off with fireworks.

I insisted the party go on. The tradition had to continue.

Was anyone in my circle really going to argue with me? I came home from the hospital weighing 11 pounds less than when I went in four days earlier.

I sat in the backyard for a while and even tried a glass of champagne, but that didn't go well. I was so desperate for the denial to kick in. I went upstairs to lie down. Lots of kids came over to play. Ava apparently sat outside, crying.

Meanwhile, I was upstairs in the bedroom. I knew that the pathology report would come through soon, very likely confirming the doctor's diagnosis. Tamara was there too. She had been so good and kind, providing me with information along the way; yet so much fell in her lap, so much terrible stuff to share. The kind of stuff my young doctor colleagues back at St.

190

Vincent's never wanted to share with their patients in dire straits.

I don't remember the fireworks.

And then – foggy and fragmented again – it was the next day, same room, twenty years to the day that Brad Hallberg and Sarah Dran had tied the knot, and now he and Mom were in the room with me, and then Tamara was there, with Ti the oncologist, who happened to live down the street.

"You have the Dana Reeve disease," Ti said. Dana Reeve had been the wife of Christopher "Superman" Reeve.

"Don't tell me that!" I said. "She's dead."

It was official. Yes, indeed. I had lung cancer.

Ti sat on the bed, trying to be both straightforward and kind. And just as in the hospital I had pressured Ti to agree that it *could* be a fungal infection, I now pressured him to say that I could survive five years. I had so much more to do. First and foremost, continuing to be a mother for as long as humanly possible, helping my kids build the resilience they would need when their mom was no longer there.

But I also had to hang around to continue my fight against the status quo in healthcare. The ten-week results of our trial had been published a few months earlier; the patients receiving the Virta treatment not only reduced their A1c levels, meaning their blood sugar was under much better control,[37] but they also experienced significant weight loss. This happened even as most of them either reduced or stopped their diabetic medications entirely. We were working on the

---

[37] See the Glossary for details about A1c.

paper for the one-year results, and we were just a few months from the end of two years.

In all the horribleness, there was a glimmer of hope. Something to distract us. Something to root for. Ti was waiting for the analysis to come back, to get more details. "You almost have to have a mutation," he said, "given that you've never smoked. As far as taking care of you, all our eggs are in that basket. If you have the mutation, then there are new treatment options that you probably don't know about."

That part was right: I didn't know. It had been years since I had been in primary care, and I wasn't well-read in oncology. I had been immersed in obesity medicine and diabetes reversal, so I was mostly in the dark about new cancer treatments – targeted therapies and immunotherapy.

I held onto something, anything. You have to. Without hope, there's nothing.

~

While we waited for the analysis I did yet more research. The norm for people in my situation was death in a very short period of time, but for some of those with specific mutations, there were stories of people living a longer time. I learned about a targeted therapy available for certain mutations, even before I knew if I had it. I started considering – and in some cases pursuing – highly experimental treatments, the kind of "solution" I would normally have rejected for its lack of scientific support. Desperate times and all that.

I read about a treatment in Cuba, a drug that was available only there, so for a few days I fixated on going to Cuba. I emailed the people in charge of the treatment. The Cuban idea fell through, a dead end, like so many other potential treatments I would pursue during the course of my disease. I didn't qualify, or it was still experimental, or the timing was off, or the treatment was still in the mice stage, and on and on. All so frustrating, but I kept searching.

We had visitors. A stream of Virta colleagues passed through. While those who had moved to Lafayette for an extended period had now all moved back home, they still came to town regularly to meet with trial patients. They came now to see me, be with me, bring us meals. One Virta pal named Camy brought a poster signed by everyone in the company.

I appreciated the attention and caring but my restlessness drained me. I had to get back to work, regardless of my diagnosis. I had to show everyone – my kids, Brad, Mom, friends, doctors, Virta colleagues, patients – that I was going to be okay, even if facts said I very probably was not.

There was a long-ago scheduled conference call with Indiana's lieutenant governor, Suzanne Crouch, and former Senator and Governor from Nebraska, Bob Kerrey, now a Virta advisor, about potentially partnering with the state to offer a path to diabetes reversal to its employees. At the time I was the main contact, and I insisted that the meeting not change. No offense, but no one at the company at the time could provide the overview I could, talking about the science, the trial, and patient care.

Even though people were nervous about my fielding the call, again: who was going to fight me on it? I kept it together for the call – and as soon as it was done, I told Brad, "I want to start taking care of patients again."

It had been barely a week since brain surgery. While we waited for word about the mutation, my cancer was growing in me. In my brain. In my lungs. We were doing nothing. When I next spoke to the oncologist, I said, "So we're just waiting for this to kill me?"

"Why don't we start chemo or radiation now for a little bit until the analysis comes back," he said.

"Let's do that," I told him. "*Now.*" I had rejected the idea in the hospital, but every patient reserves the right to completely change her mind.

The phone rang the next morning. I could see it was Ti.

"You have the mutation we were hoping for," he said.

~ ~ ~

Chapter 17

Making the Best

Now I had a little hope – hope is hope.

I would be getting an infusion every three weeks plus "targeted therapy" in pill form. It's targeted because it is not indiscriminate like other chemotherapies which attack all cells. Instead, it zeroes in on the pathway of growth needed, in my case, by my mutation.

Our hope was that this one-two punch would basically suffocate the tumor, with my immune system doing its part to help. I was excited. There was a plan.

"They can mail you the pill and you'll have it in two days," said Ti.

Two days? I'd already gone a week doing nothing to slow the tumor's growth.

"No, no, no, I'm not waiting two days," I said, my usual impatient self. "Where's it being shipped from?"

Ti named a lab in Indianapolis. I asked him to call and tell them I was on my way to pick it up that day.

Brad and I drove to Indy, I jumped out of the car as soon as he pulled up, and sprinted into the building. Waiting in the lobby was someone from the lab with my pills. I untwisted the bottle and downed my first dose, right there in the middle of the lobby. If I'd been in a different mood, I might have laughed at how the scene looked: an intense woman making a weird drug exchange in a very public place, crazed for her fix.

~

By month's end, just four weeks after brain surgery, I had returned to work, running group classes at the clinic. Nobody fought with me very much about returning though I think everybody thought it was a dumb idea. But that's who I was. That was my way of coping – jump right back in, an attempt to be the old me, the healthy me.

I felt bad that I was less involved than I wanted in writing the paper on the trial's one-year results for those with diabetes, but I did lots of editing. The results were exciting. We started with 262 adults with diabetes in the experimental group. Most were on diabetes medications, and most were obese (average BMI was 40.[38]). They had lived with diabetes an average of 8.4 years and many were on insulin. Many nutrition studies of people with diabetes include only the newly diagnosed and often do not include those on insulin. We had the tough cases.

After one year, 218 patients were still in the experimental group; in the world of clinical trials, that 83% retention rate is an amazing feat for a lifestyle program. Our ongoing remote care model – health coaches, monitors, apps, and daily communication – encouraged and enabled adherence. Continuous care was also necessary because the often-rapid declines in blood sugar required rapid changes in medications.

---

[38] Body Mass Index. A BMI of 25 to 30 is overweight, 30 and above are considered obese. See the Glossary for the calculation of BMI.

Blood sugar levels were down and there was less variability in the levels over time. A remarkable 60% of the remaining participants reversed their diabetes. Ninety-four percent of the participants who started the trial on insulin therapy reduced or eliminated it altogether. Although weight loss was not the main goal of the study, after that first year participants averaged 12% loss of body weight (average of 30 pounds!). Liver function improved. Markers for inflammation were down. Of the 26 markers for cardiovascular disease (CVD), 22 decreased.[39] (Type 2 diabetes is a known risk factor for CVD.) There were *no* adverse effects attributable to the treatment.

In the control group, there were no significant decreases in A1c, weight, or use of diabetes medication; *and none of them reversed their diabetes.*[40]

~

---

[39] Most notably, there was reduction in blood pressure, reduction in triglycerides, decrease in the triglyceride/HDL-C ratio, and increase in HDL-C. There was an increase in LDL-C in some participants (See the Glossary for details. See also Chapter 8, pages 104-105 for details about the relationships among saturated fat, LDL, and cardiovascular risk). Details of the discussion on cardiovascular risk are in: Bhanpuri NH, Hallberg SJ, Williams PT, McKenzie AL, Ballard KD, Campbell WW, McCarter JP, Phinney SD, Volek JS. "Cardiovascular Disease Risk Factor Responses to a Type 2 Diabetes Care Model Including Nutritional Ketosis Induced by Sustained Carbohydrate Restriction at One Year: An Open Label, Non-Randomized, Controlled Study." *Cardiovascular Diabetology.* **17**, Article number: 56 (2018). cardiab.biomedcentral.com/articles/10.1186/s12933-018-0698-8

[40] After a year, one of the control patients called the clinic office, upset and chastising the staff — she had friends in the experimental group and they were getting better while she wasn't.

As for when I *wasn't* at work? It was tough going from being a provider in a medical network to a patient. There were the looks I got walking into the oncology clinic. At times I had the curtains closed around my seated self during an infusion, just like any patient. One of my patients just had to see for herself. "Dr. Sarah!" she exclaimed, as she poked her head in. "Oh my god, I can't believe it's Dr. Sarah!"

I began a coast-to-coast odyssey, visiting cancer centers with specialists in my mutation. An appointment at a major cancer hospital in New York City, where doctors were working on new therapies, turned out to be a dead end, but I couldn't help but feel my privilege; how fortunate (and unfair) that I could find out about these possible therapies because of my connections in the medical world, while most people with cancer don't have that access.

It was one of many realities of health inequity that I would absorb even more deeply once I became a patient. What about the less well-positioned? Try this, for an example:

A 36-year-old single mother of three works full-time as an administrative assistant at a very small business, plus part-time as a customer service phone representative. Both jobs are not far from her home, which is a good thing because she can't afford a car, and must walk to work every day. She relies on a patchwork of financial help from family, along with some government-supported child care. Does any of this sound outlandish? Like anyone you know? Like your own life? Although this woman's children are a healthy weight, she herself has gained a lot over the past five years. The stress of a divorce and being a single parent causes her often to feel overwhelmed. She has virtually no time to worry about herself, though, so when she starts having stomach pain, she doesn't think too much about it. The pain gets worse.

Let's say this woman has health insurance; then again, her deductible seems financially out of reach right now. Last year she had to take her daughter to the Emergency Room for an asthma attack and wound up with a huge bill that she's still paying off. She just can't take on another debt like that. But then she starts bleeding and gets dizzy and falls at work. She feels so weak that she cannot resist when her co-workers call 911.

In the ER she is found to be extremely anemic, and has a large tumor in her colon and several smaller tumors in her liver. Colon cancer, stage 4. She is assigned a patient navigator who helps make sure she has the right appointments and even assists her in figuring out disability coverage. She has to have surgery, then chemo. She misses a lot of work. When her Family and Medical Leave times are over, she's fired.

I may be making up this example but it's anything but fantasy.

The woman cannot make ends meet with disability insurance so as soon as she's done with chemo, she finds a new job. Two years go by and things seem back to "normal." Then she develops a cough. By the time she's able to find a "free" hour to get to the doctor, she's coughing up blood. The cancer is back.

When cancer returns, there is often no patient navigator around to help. It is as if recurrence is a different disease, a less pressing one (if pressing at all).

Gone are the quick procedures and appointments. Gone, often, is the urgency. There are standard treatments for recurrence, but often, especially for young patients, a clinical trial may be the best option. This woman is poor. She has no reliable transportation. The closest appropriate trial location is eight hours away and not in her network. She is lucky that her oncologist even discusses a trial with her! Many doctors simply don't, especially when they know that the finances are likely to overwhelm the patient.

The woman begins to lose hope.

Hope is something promoted for only some patients. This woman is not one of them. She dies from cancer less than a year later.

Would this have happened if she were in a higher financial class and had a support system? Almost certainly the outcome would have been different.

~

A couple weeks after beginning targeted therapy, I had another lung scan. Every tumor was gone except for the primary, which had shrunk by 60%. Brad and I texted all our friends. Everyone came over that night and we had a party. We drank champagne. Brad and I always kept a bottle of champagne in the refrigerator. We didn't open one very often but I believed that if you didn't have champagne chilling in the fridge, then you didn't expect something good to happen. I didn't want to live like that.

Hope. The difference between living without hope and living with it is . . . well, everything.

~

In the meantime I'd committed to giving a lecture at a national obesity meeting in San Antonio. You can't do everything, but apparently I never got the memo to stop trying. For the last several years, I had gotten in the habit of saying yes to everything, and it was not a habit easily broken, lung cancer or no. I felt blessed to be involved in such an exciting medical field, where things were truly changing, and I couldn't help but feel that conditions were never going to be exactly like this again. So I went to Texas.

Traveling while undergoing cancer treatment is something I would probably advise against. (If you can't hear the sarcasm in that sentence: It's sarcastic. *Very*.) It seemed as if for every other conference I attended I forgot to pack essential things, like clothes, so I would hunt down the local TJ Maxx or equivalent to buy a dress or two. That aspect of chemo, the brain fog, could seem almost charming, though. No, the part that was so tough was just . . . moving. Walking. Standing. Smiling. Pretending. By the time I was heading home, whether I had been gone for three days or less than 24 hours, shuffling through the airport to my gate seemed like a marathon. I felt depleted and sad and alone, hiding a terrible secret, as I looked at all the healthy people (or seemingly healthy people). I hated how briskly everyone passed me, even men and women in their 70s. Their 80s?

Were the walls of the massive airport terminal closing in on everyone else the way they seemed to be on me?

Was every seat and bench I passed really calling

out my name, *Sarah, come, sit, take a nap, Sarah?*
Why had I packed my suitcase with bricks?

~

Before my diagnosis my diet was ketogenic; I continued to follow it even as I was unsure that it had any real effect on my situation. Early studies showed promising results for cancer patients on a ketogenic diet. Unfortunately, the one cancer that so far appeared unresponsive to diet was lung cancer. Basically, if you have lung cancer, it doesn't seem to matter what the hell you eat.

I was losing a lot of weight. But putting on weight was difficult because I had nausea every day. I switched to a plain old whole-food diet, and still had trouble digesting protein. I couldn't tolerate meat, cheese, most things. Vegetables and fruit (mostly berries) were the only foods I could really keep down, my primary calorie and energy source – not a great strategy for gaining weight. I got some protein from peanut butter. I had trouble with other nuts. I couldn't tolerate much of anything anymore.

~

By this time I was completely bald and began wearing a wig, a common enough practice in that situation, I was pretending something was that wasn't. I was in denial, desperate to hide my diagnosis. By that point in my professional life I had antagonized lots of people because of the research our team and I had been doing, and I had made lots of enemies for the things I was saying publicly. The ADA had not liked my TEDx talk. Some of the most vocal members of the vegan community felt that I was pushing meat (untrue). My *New York Times* op-ed recommending a change of diet before resorting to potentially dangerous and expensive surgery did not go over well with bariatric surgeons or the ADA. The status quo people did not want the American population listening to me. (I know that sounds grandiose but I believe it's true.) If any of my adversaries knew I had cancer, it could make their social media bashing of me worse.

~

How do you slow down when that's never, ever been your speed? And you're a 46-year-old woman who until very recently put in 60+-hour work weeks, was the principal investigator for a large clinical trial, and was, along with her husband, raising three children? And who worked out multiple times a week? And who drank from the fire hose at all times?

A few months before I was diagnosed I found myself in a circle of some of my closest friends, and the conversation turned to furniture. One friend said she had a favorite chair and described what she loved about it. Someone else talked about her favorite chair and its appeal, then another one about hers. I didn't want to be the wet blanket but when it was my turn, I said, "I know people have their favorite chairs but honestly . . . I guess I've never had one. I don't know what a favorite chair would be."

Tamara looked at me like I was from Mars. "Sarah, you don't have a favorite chair," she said, "because you've never sat down long enough for any chair to *be* your favorite."

For most of my life, I had run as hard as I could, all the time. That was me. That was who everyone knew as me.

Now what?

~   ~   ~

Chapter 18

Getting the Word Out

I was back leading groups at IUH. Quite a few of our patients had grown attached to me; I felt as if I were a surrogate therapist for them. What they didn't realize was that my helping them was helping me. It was giving me another purpose and that felt good.

I never stopped working during chemo and, maybe even more importantly, I never stopped traveling for work. How could I? We were doing something amazing in health care. The study was going great and we had to educate as many people about it as we could. I was good at communicating our results and answering questions. It was best done live, so I attended conferences and meetings of all kinds.

One of those trips was to a large American Indian Nation in Oklahoma. The experience performed double duty: Britt and I met with employees of the Nation, plus Noah joined us, a way for mom and son to spend time together, and to let him see first-hand why I was fussing so much about diabetes care.

The toll on Indigenous Americans from poor nutrition and the consequent illnesses, especially diabetes, is staggering. According to the CDC, American Indians have the highest rate of diabetes of any racial or ethnic group in the country, about twice that of the White population. Unless the trend is halted, one in two American Indian children will eventually become diabetic. Most American Indians on reservations live in food deserts, where the only grocery store or market is at best many miles away and where much of their sustenance comes from the USDA's Food Distribution Program, which consists largely of high-carbohydrate and processed foods. Enter diabetes, an illness for which Indigenous American languages did not even have a word.

We met with representatives of the Nation's employees and with some of their members who were being treated for diabetes. We talked to them about the science of what we were doing and how to reduce or eliminate drugs in their treatment of diabetes. The trip led to one of Virta's early contracts.

It was so important to me, so gratifying, that our message was reaching people who were typically among the last to be thought about.

~

When we came out with our one-year trial results in February 2018, the mainstream media ignored us, although politico.com gave a brief write-up. They quoted an executive from a health IT company, who said that if this were a drug, "it would be the biggest blockbuster in history."

I had a great conversation with Mark Hyman for his podcast, *The Doctor's Farmacy*, where we talked at length about – as he titled it – "The Ground-Breaking Study You Haven't Heard About." He said more or less the same thing the health IT executive said; when our results were published, Dr. Hyman had expected a front-page story touting the "greatest breakthrough in science in 100 years." He was shocked when, instead, only one newspaper, *The Detroit News*, picked it up. And the only reason *they* covered it was because I had written an op-ed about the study which they published. That piece began with the sentence, "Diabetes is reversible."[41] You'd think that would have garnered some attention, no? The disease that defines maybe the biggest health epidemic of the last generation, the present generation, and the next one – and it's *reversible*? My second sentence: "That's the exciting conclusion of a study I'm leading at Indiana University Health." You'd think *that* would make people even more curious and excited – that my conclusion was based on scientific evidence!

Nope.

Never mind my article had stated that the science was clear that reversing diabetes was possible; never mind that we now had a reasonable, exciting path to achieving the goal of diabetes reversal through a healthy diet: the mainstream press ignored our one-year study.

Fortunately, I was soon flooded with speaking invitations from groups that were themselves studying or promoting low-carb diets and approaches to weight loss or diabetes reversal through diet. They understood that our study was moving the goalposts. It was so satisfying to get this kind of attention. It wasn't so long ago that our research about low-carb and diabetes reversal and insulin deprescription was met with almost

---

[41] "Don't manage diabetes, reverse it." *The Detroit News*, June 5, 2018. detroitnews.com/story/opinion/2018/06/05/opinion-dont-manage-diabetes-reverse/670756002/

complete silence, from nearly all corners; I had desperately wanted to get calls asking me to come talk about our work and its implications. Eager to get the word out, I would have gone anywhere and talked to anyone – anyone! – who expressed interest.

Now that wish was starting to be realized, at least from segments of the scientific-medical-nutrition communities. Each week brought multiple inquiries. *Can you come speak at our conference? Do you have time for a phone interview?* I said yes to nearly everything. I traveled often. It was a ridiculous, exhausting schedule, but I wanted so badly to promote our important work, and feel relevant, to feel that I still had a purpose.

~

People often talk about bucket lists, special things they want to do or see before they die. Mine? I was going to have to work extra fast to fill it. So the whole family went to Belize. We snorkeled. We spent time in the jungle. Growing up in the Midwest, seeing a jungle had been on my bucket list.

Check.

Next on the list: hiking the Inca Trail to Machu Picchu. Probably not a great idea for someone with lung cancer who recently underwent chest radiation. Not only that but shortly before we left for Peru, I started having chest pains. I told no one about the pain, not even Brad. Once there, I did better than I expected. Though I was the slowest in my group, by far, our guide told me I was faster than average. Still, I was in a private panic about the pain; as my mind raced through the possibilities, I periodically consoled myself with this admittedly morbid thought: *Hey, if you're gonna die, what a beautiful place to do it.*

After a few days there the pain started to diminish. There are few joys as thrilling and deep as the one where you're certain that you're feeling noticeably better – or noticeably less unwell. I kept my excitement to myself but it was hard. I was determined not to "talk cancer" on the trip. The pain, it would turn out, was a delayed reaction to the radiation.

Machu Picchu. Check.

My family flew home while I continued on to Zurich for an international nutrition conference titled "Food for Thought: The Science and Politics of Nutrition," hosted by Swiss Re Institute, the research arm of Swiss Re, an insurance company that insures other insurance companies. Swiss Re was exploring ways to deal with "a chronic epidemic of non-communicable diseases" – cardiovascular, cancers, respiratory, and especially diabetes. Insurance companies have every incentive to want to reduce the incidence of these diseases, which is good for the rest of us too. Swiss Re estimated that the annual world bill for diabetes treatment was over $1,000,000,000,000. That's one trillion dollars. In 2017, the yearly US bill for diabetes and its effects, including lost productivity, was well over $300 billion.[42]

---

[42] Editor's note: as of 2023, the yearly bill for diabetes and its effects, including lost productivity, is well over $400 billion. American Diabetes Association, Press Release. "New American Diabetes Association Report Finds Annual Costs of Diabetes to be $412.9 Billion." diabetes.org/newsroom/press-releases/new-american-diabetes-association-report-finds-annual-costs-diabetes-be

I took part in a panel discussion on "Low Carb High-Fat Diets: Public Controversies and Opportunities," moderated by Fiona Godlee, editor-in-chief of *The BMJ,* one of the world's top-ranked medical journals (formerly *The British Medical Journal*). There were definitely controversies among members of the panel and thoughtful questions from the audience. My principal messages, which garnered broad agreement, was that reversal, not just management, should be a goal of type 2 diabetes treatment; that patients should be made aware of that goal; and that they should know the choices available to them in reaching the goal – bariatric surgery, restricted calories, or carbohydrate restriction (low-carb or ketogenic diet). Several of those in the audience – mostly doctors, researchers, and nutritionists – were themselves already following a low-carb lifestyle.

Of course, I couldn't resist pushing back on flimsy, dangerous thinking. When one audience member asserted that Asians who moved to Britain started having problems with diabetes and heart disease, cancer, and kidney stones because they were eating more meat and fat than before they had emigrated, I blurted out, "Based on what data?" Fiona Godlee politely silenced me. But my point: people often jump to conclusions when they see such a change, like an increase in health problems among immigrants. There is no evidence that meat is the cause. On the other hand, there's plenty of evidence to show that sugar and processed foods are major culprits, and perhaps the "overeating," including greater carb consumption, that is common in Western societies.

During the previous year I had appeared on so many podcasts that it felt almost as if they were following me around. In fact, that's what happened in Zurich, where I was approached by two men who did a podcast titled *2 Keto Dudes* who asked did I want to be on their show? Of course I said yes. I appreciated how they zeroed in on my defense of the average person's ability to stick with a low-carb diet, and the high retention rate (83% after the first year) that we had shown in our study.

~

Big fall trip to Washington, DC, and the Capitol. I presented the costs, both human and financial, of diabetes in the US, as well as the results of our one-year trial, to "The Food Is Medicine" Working Group, a part of the bipartisan House Hunger Caucus. Its purpose is to study nutrition policy for improving the health of Americans and consequently reducing health costs resulting from poor diet. We brought one of our patients – so fit and healthy looking – to tell of his experiences with our program. The only problem he had had with losing weight, he said, was that none of his clothes fit him anymore. Frankly, I don't think my presentation had an impact – yet. But we keep nibbling away at the status quo by getting our message out far and wide. Congress was one of many places to nibble.

Once again, my trip served a double purpose. Noah and Ava came along and got to see the amazing Smithsonian National Museum of African American History and Culture, a wonderful educational stop, plus enjoy a Southern lunch (good food). They also got to eat breakfast in a Congressional cafeteria (food not so good, and lots of carbs).

Soon after we returned home, *The Hill*, a political news site, published an op-ed of mine titled "Government Dietary Guidelines Are Plain Wrong: Avoid Carbs, Not Fat." [43] It was a plea for the government to pay more attention to recent research about the health effects of fats versus carbohydrates.

Meanwhile, our research, our focus on improving the Virta continuous care process, our interacting with patients and encouraging colleagues: all of that was vitally important. But maybe my most critical role now was promoting our work, letting the general public and the medical/nutrition world (or those in that world willing to listen) know that *evidence showed diabetes is reversible through diet*. I would do everything in my power not to let that life-altering fact be ignored.

In late 2019, everyone still in the Virta trial had completed three and a half years; out of the original 262 patients with diabetes, 143 (54.6%) were still with us. (The study ended after two years for the control patients.) Some patients with diabetes chose not to continue after two years, the majority of those because of some life crisis, or because they simply decided they no longer wanted to participate. To retain over half the participants after three-plus years was truly extraordinary.

It was not only patients who had been living with

---

[43] "Government Dietary Guidelines Are Plain Wrong: Avoid Carbs, Not Fat." *The Hill*, November 29, 2018.
thehill.com/opinion/healthcare/419020-government-dietary-guidelines-are-plain-wrong-avoid-carbs-not-fat

diabetes for a short time who were successful. Remember, we had the tough cases. And during those three years, three of our patients who had been living with diabetes the longest – 15 to 20 years, and on huge doses of insulin – came completely off their insulin. More than three years in the trial and they stuck with it! They needed proper food. *We* need proper food. It works. I can only imagine how much money people with diabetes and their insurance companies will save.

I was back on chemo and feeling the effects. Still, I had committed to giving a presentation in Lansing at Michigan State University, College of Human Medicine, on "Reversing Type 2 Diabetes: Change the Paradigm and Change Lives." There was to be a dinner the evening before, breakfast the day of, and the presentation at noon. The dinner was the first thing I canceled; just too tired. Then the breakfast got scratched, same reason. Then my flight there. I just didn't see how I could make it. I was at the kitchen counter with my laptop open to a map showing the location of the talk when my mom stopped by. I told her how badly I felt about canceling. She looked at the map.

"It's only a four-hour drive," she said. "I'll take you."

(Had I just conned my mom?!)

I took another nap and we left. While she drove and listened to the audiobook of *Becoming* by Michelle Obama, I slept. At the hotel I went straight to bed. The next morning I actually felt awake and the presentation went fine – well, except for one thing. Prior to the talk I had cut my finger. Just a little. The tiniest thing really, which would otherwise have gone unnoticed, including by me . . . except I was on blood thinner. The cut soon bled through the Band-Aid. And down my finger. And onto the podium. I had to alter my usual presentation style – arms and hands animated – or blood would be flying everywhere. I felt handicapped at not being able to flap and gesture.

Afterwards I had a conversation with Dr. Saleh Aldasouqi, Head of the Division of Endocrinology and Metabolism at MSU, who had invited me to speak. We discussed our mutual, passionate interest in and concerns about *pre*-prediabetes. Pre-prediabetes is not often considered; it's really an emerging concept – but it's the beginning of the road to type 2 diabetes. During this time, the body is working hard to keep blood sugar and insulin at normal levels. Dr. Aldasouqi and I both felt that before we started to see the markers for prediabetes and diabetes – A1c and fasting blood sugar – we should be more attentive to individuals who exhibit any signs they're heading down this path, especially increased weight and most especially waist circumference, a significant risk factor for type 2 diabetes.[44] That attention could help many people head off development of prediabetes and then full-blown diabetes. At this time there are no recommended routine tests to identify pre-prediabetes. But thinking and talking about it are the precursors for change.

We also discussed that endocrinologists usually see insulin as a miracle drug (clearly it is for those with type 1 diabetes or a damaged pancreas), to the point that they can be slow to consider other treatments, such as reducing carbohydrate intake (which would, of course, mean "ignoring the guidelines").

---

[44] See the Glossary for details.

On the way home, I was awake enough to catch a little of Michelle.

~

All this time, we continued the Virta webinars. Sometimes they were for patients, sometimes current Virta clients, sometimes potential clients. Members of our web audience were able to interact with questions and comments. Although the webinars worked well, I didn't feel quite the same thrill I had when I was in the room with my colleagues and the audience. I would be in Indiana while Britt was in New Jersey. Or I would be in my kitchen while Dr. Shaminie Athinarayanan, a Virta researcher and first author or co-author of dozens of our publications, was across town. Later, when Covid-19 struck, webinars would be a vital part of our repertoire.

My own health odyssey was, as cancer odysseys almost always are, at once epic and banal. As personal as it gets, and, sadly, so similar to what too many people are experiencing at that exact moment. Anyone who has been through it knows all too well that there are more periods of pain, distress, and despair than you would ever want to recount, including to yourself, and I won't chronicle anywhere close to all of mine. But some moments stand out, especially because they so directly impacted other moments. In the fall of 2019, while in San Francisco for a Virta offsite business/team-building event, I felt shortness of breath. I was so fatigued that after dinner Tamara and Britt had to push me for a block because it was uphill. I felt like a piece of furniture, maybe a piece of furniture with shuffling feet. They pushed, I shuffled. If anyone was observing the scene from across the street, I wonder what they made of the three of us.

By the time I returned home, the shortness of breath was extreme enough that I wound up in the hospital, diagnosed with atypical hemolytic uremic syndrome, which has a 50% mortality rate in the first few days. The chances of getting this from my particular chemo was 0.6% – about 1 in every 165 people – and then only after being on it for four to seven months. I'd been on it for all of four weeks. I didn't call myself "The Queen of Side Effects" for nothing. I experienced kidney failure. And liver failure. And respiratory failure. And viral pneumonia. And, likely, interstitial pneumonitis. The statistical probability of getting all of these at once is basically zero.

Somehow – you probably guessed – I didn't die. Not yet. I got home from the hospital in time for my 48th birthday. After weeks of treatment, my kidneys recovered.

Gradually, I started doing more work. I did an interview for a documentary titled *Fat Fiction*, directed by Jennifer Isenhart and executive-produced by Amanda Atkins (no relation to the Atkins diet), who has also produced a horror film. How appropriate, because *Fat Fiction* is a nutrition horror story. It tells the tale that I had been trying to tell, and continued trying to tell. It's the story of how, without evidence, we were sold on a diet – low-fat and high carb – that not only was unhealthy but brought untold misery and death. The film presents data on the increasing rates of obesity and diabetes over the past several decades. If a picture is worth a thousand words, then a few video clips are positively mind-blowing. I'm talking about random street scenes from 40-50 years ago (Who are all those slender people?) and then from today (Why are so many people overweight or obese?). The comedian and social critic Bill Maher summed it up after viewing a clip of onlookers at the 1969 launch of Apollo XI: "I was struck by how not fat everyone in the crowd was. We look like a completely different race of people."

But *Fat Fiction*[45] is also a story of hope. In addition to the scientific explanations and a history of the American diet, it tracks three healthy individuals who follow a ketogenic diet for one week and then a low-fat diet recommended by the Guidelines for a week. During the ketogenic week all three individuals recorded low, steady blood sugar levels (they were supplied with a blood sugar monitoring patch and an app to record it on their phones). They were not hungry between meals; they each lost weight. During Week 2, the low-fat diet week, a graph of blood sugar recordings looked like a roller coaster and spiked higher; they were often hungry, and not as energetic.

And then there was the story of the military helicopter pilot who was forced to stop flying because of an unknown illness – until he stopped eating a by-the-Guidelines, military-recommended diet and switched to a low-carb diet. The happy ending: he felt great and returned to flying. There are more happy-ending stories documented in the film.

Of course, these are anecdotes, not hard evidence. But they put faces, very human, everyday

---

[45] *Fat Fiction* is a full-length documentary and can be seen on YouTube.

faces, on what evidence-based nutrition science has been telling us.

A popular podcast, Kara Swisher's *Recode Decode*, invited me to talk about Virta and entrepreneurship in Indiana. My state and the Midwest in general are not usually associated with innovation and tech. At conferences where I talked about our advances in telehealth, I had grown accustomed to comments like, "Indiana? Who knew?" But there was quite a bit going on in "flyover" country. Given the techy focus of *Recode Decode*, they were especially interested in the innovative way that we at Virta were using telemedicine, with monitors and apps, to communicate with and encourage patients, and the great success we were having with it. It wasn't many years ago that this would have been considered Star Trek crazy stuff.

Then I was lucky enough and grateful to the ADA for letting me speak about the science *against* "you are what you eat," at their first-ever virtual Annual Meeting in 2020. My argument centered around the word "fat." You do *not* get fat because you eat fat. When you eat fat – instead of so many carbohydrates – your body is fueled primarily by the fat. It is not stored in those fat cells. The old idea behind "you are what you eat" was simple (simplistic and wrong): cut the fat out of your diet, you're going to cut the fat out of you.

No. Not the same thing. The confusion no doubt goes back to the word "fat" as food and "fat" on the body. Remember how I wanted to include in my TEDx talk that the confusion between dietary fat and body fat might be avoided "if we just called dietary fat something else, like rainbows and butterflies"?

Vindicated!

~   ~   ~

218

Chapter 19

Bye Bye, Low Fat

From the beginning, Virta's message was one filled with hope. Happily, excitingly, our results validated that hope, and each year was more persuasive (and hopeful!) than the last. Our trial started in 2015 and we were psyched and thrilled about the first-year results we published early in 2018.

In June 2019, we published our two-year results. Retention for the treatment group was 74%, again an amazing number for a lifestyle change in a clinical trial, attesting to the effectiveness of continuous remote care. Our patients experienced sustained improvements in A1c, fasting blood sugar, blood pressure, triglycerides, inflammation, liver function, and weight; HDL, the good cholesterol, increased. The control group had no improvements in these markers.

After the two years, 53.5% had diabetes reversal and 17.6% had what the ADA considers remission, partial or complete.[46] There continued to be no adverse effects attributable to the treatment.

In the control group there were no reversals and 2.4% partial remission.

---

[46] In reversal, diabetes medicines are eliminated except possibly metformin. In remission metformin is also eliminated and there are some criteria for the length of time without medication.

And let's not forget the participants who were prediabetic. They received the same treatments as the diabetic participants but were analyzed separately. After two years, 75% were still in the program. Only 3% had gone on to type 2 diabetes and 52.3% had reversed out of prediabetes (they now had A1c below 5.7% without medication). Other biomarkers improved, including weight loss. We compared these results with other studies for the prevention or delay of progression to type 2 diabetes. Our two-year patient retention rate was far higher; more patients had weight loss of 5% or more; there was a much higher incidence of backing out of prediabetes, and lower progression to type 2 diabetes.

The trial concluded in spring 2021 after five amazing years,[47] the longest such trial to date. We had followed a protocol as rigorous as had ever been done in a diet trial. We had been blessed with a cohort that was not only significant in number, but so many of our original participants had stayed with the program throughout those five years – 46.6% of the original diabetic patients, a remarkable number for a lifestyle study. That helped make our evidence powerful, able to stand up to scrutiny.[48] All along, Virta was putting out a stream of videos on YouTube that answered questions about low-carb/high-fat and how the Virta approach worked. I appeared in several of them, sometimes with Britt, sometimes with Steve, sometimes with others. I

---

[47] The trial started in August of 2015 and ended in late April 2021, five plus years. Completing patients each participated for five years, but their ending dates depended on when they enrolled between August 2015 and April 2016.

[48] By early 2022, the results for various aspects of the trial had already appeared in a dozen publications.

have to admit that these were a step (or two) up from the amateur videos Brad and I had once produced in our living room.

The company expanded.[49] Many of the contracts are with self-insured employers, which means they pay the medical costs of their employees. Why so many self-insured? The cost of the Virta program is less than their medical bills have been. It's pretty simple: employees who are not sick (or less sick) cost less.

We were not the only ones pounding away at paradigms that were false and dangerous ("diabetes is not reversible," "saturated fat is bad," etc.). You could feel a real shift in communities that were focused on nutrition, obesity, diabetes, and overall health and well-being, brave thinkers willing to question a status quo that had been failing miserably for so long. Lots of research and advocacy was coming from other supporters of carbohydrate restriction for metabolic health, including reversing type 2 diabetes, and for a generally healthy lifestyle. Increasingly, there were indications that news of the accumulating scientific evidence was focused squarely on the public: an explosion of podcasts and YouTube videos aimed at a general audience discussed low carb. It was thrilling to field so many requests for interviews, podcasts, panels, and conferences.

Often it's something small and personal that shows just how much an idea has finally permeated the culture. One day Mom was shopping in a Lafayette grocery store when she overheard this father-and-son

---

[49] Editor's note: By the end of 2022, Virta had partnered with more than 350 large employers, health plans, and government organizations, including Humana, Banner|Aetna, U-Haul, and AutoZone.

exchange:

Son: "Are carbs healthy?"

Dad: "Well, some of them. But if you have too much, no."

After recounting the story, Mom said, "You had something to do with that, Sarah."

I felt like crying.

I was not alone in the fight, not even close, especially given all the amazing pioneers and status quo-fighters on whose work our own was building. We had come a long way and it was, and always is, important to reflect on the positive markers along the road. Looking back, some moments particularly stood out to me. In 2018, at the Swiss Re/BMJ "Food for Thought" conference in Zurich, I witnessed a remarkable push against low-fat as a healthy diet. The closing statement from Fiona Godlee, editor-in-chief of *The BMJ*, included the exhortation, to an audience of experts, that nutrition science needed to be open to new evidence, which might mean admitting you were wrong. Seen against the backdrop of some of the entrenched thinking (and thinkers) we had been fighting, it was an astonishing statement, and such a welcome one. Godlee focused on the unfounded vilification of saturated fat.

That was a moment.

There was also the acknowledgment – though a long time coming – from some of the most influential organizations in their fields. For starters, as I've noted, back in 2016 the ADA had endorsed bariatric surgery as a therapeutic option for treating type 2 diabetes. Credit to them for that shift – away from disease management only – but they didn't go further and mention the potential and profound benefits of a low-carb diet.

Then, after years of the ADA's doctors and spokespeople ridiculing or ignoring the massive benefits of the low-carb diet, even warning that consuming fewer than 130 grams of carbohydrates a day is actually dangerous, the 2018 ADA/EASD (European Association for the Study of Diabetes) joint statement listed a low-carb diet as a blood sugar-lowering therapy, a real turning point. Not the robust recommendation we would have liked, but it was still a breakthrough. The 2019 ADA Nutrition Therapy Consensus Report and Standards of Medical Care went on to recommend that practitioners offer their diabetes patients individual nutrition options, including low-carb choices. That report also acknowledged that medications can be reduced with a low-carb diet. And in 2020, the ADA came out with its strongest-ever endorsement for the low-carb diet, citing three of our papers. Very exciting.

The AHA – among the first health organizations to embrace low-fat, especially low saturated fat, as the way to protect against cardiovascular disease, and a long-time champion of Ancel Keys' diet-heart hypothesis – was slower and more uneven in modifying its stance. That's how the status quo works. It had been closely aligned with the Dietary Guidelines for Americans, which have steadfastly ignored the research and science on carbohydrate restrictions. But along the way, the AHA began to back off its language of a low-fat diet. True, they did this in the middle of the night, metaphorically; there were no press releases noting this monumental shift. That was uncool, not to announce their altered view publicly, because it meant that except for those of us in the field, no one realized a shift in the

AHA thinking had even happened! It was the equivalent of trying slowly to back out of a room without being noticed . . . but (staying positive, embracing hope) at least they made the change. And to its credit, the AHA has gradually increased warnings about sugar, and stopped giving its "heart healthy" check-off to sugary, high-carb cereals. (Somehow, because these cereals are low in fat, the AHA had considered them "healthy," a testimony to the power of the low-fat idea.)_[50]

Though progress was slow for the ADA and the AHA, they at least moved forward. I can't say the same for those running the Dietary Guidelines for Americans. As I write this, in the fall of 2021, the Guidelines continue to ignore the evidence from low-carb research. The low-fat diet is not dead. But it is dying. I'm proud that our team is among the status quo fighters helping to push it toward the edge. There have been so many head-to-head trials of low-carb versus low-fat, and low-carb always wins. *Always.* At this point, the low-carb diet has been studied in well over 7,000 people. There are low-

---

[50] Editor's note: In January 2022 in a paragraph on nutrition in its publication, *Circulation,* the American Heart Association publicly recognized that low-carb and very low-carb diets (not defined) can lower A1c in diabetes patients, reduce the use of medications, and result in weight loss. It was not a whole-hearted endorsement, but the recognition was nonetheless groundbreaking for the AHA. Joseph JJ, Deedwania P, Acharya T, Aguilar D, Bhatt DL, Chyun DA, Di Palo KE, Golden SH, Sperling LS, on behalf of the American Heart Association Diabetes Committee of the Council on Lifestyle and Cardiometabolic Health; Council on Arteriosclerosis, Thrombosis and Vascular Biology; Council on Clinical Cardiology; and Council on Hypertension. "Comprehensive Management of Cardiovascular Risk Factors for Adults With Type 2 Diabetes: A Scientific Statement From the American Heart Association." *Circulation,* 2022;145:e722–e759. www.ahajournals.org/doi/full/10.1161/CIR.0000000000001040

carb movements in numerous countries. There is considerable funding for more research, including research on different patient demographics.

The low-fat diet is dying. We just need a final reckoning, because far too many people, including those whose health and well-being and very lives depend on this revelatory information, still don't know it.

~ ~ ~

Chapter 20

The Last Chapter

As I write this, in February 2022, I've already beaten the odds. I have done everything I know as a doctor, a scientist, and a human being to hunt down and try things that might work, or at least slow the disease. I have been open to the known (status quo) and the unknown. I have gone way past Plans B and C and D and am now deep into the alphabet.[51]

A year ago, in the winter of 2021, I visited another cancer center, looking for an answer. It was my sixth different facility. Or maybe my seventh.

I took most of the summer off. Just wanted to be with the kids. Recover mentally and physically. I was so wiped. When I told Virta I needed the time off, the support was overwhelming. "Finally! It's about time!" was the most common response.

In July I had full-brain radiation. It's as radical as it sounds. By August all my hair was gone and I could not focus for long periods – 60-hour work weeks are now a distant memory.

In the final months of 2021, I was still taking part in a clinical trial for my type of cancer. It is clear now that this one isn't going to work for me. As it became

---

[51] There are researchers out there pushing for new approaches for my particular cancer. No surprise – I tried some. They just aren't there yet.

obvious that the fight was ending, I expressed some of my thoughts in a few Facebook "essays," reflections on how I now see the world and my place in it. I have included here some edited extracts from these postings, in addition to other thoughts, both personal and professional.

Facebook
September 16, 2021

It was hard for me to shift from being a physician to a cancer patient. It was hard to switch from being a researcher to a research participant. I guess that's because when you have cancer, enrolling in a trial often means you are more than sick; you are desperate.

Despite my late-stage cancer, I am fortunate in many ways. As a physician, I can quickly absorb mounds of research literature. I have connections to answer additional questions or guidance when I need them. I had learned to be a relentless advocate for my patients, and I transferred that skill to myself.

One thing that has become devastatingly obvious to me during my cancer battle is the stark disparity in treatment options for privileged White people like myself versus disadvantaged minorities and lower-income individuals. This includes the ability to enroll in a clinical trial. Barriers to enrollment have been studied for years. Congress even legislated increasing diversity in clinical trials back in 1993. In 2014, the Food and Drug Administration set up an action plan to report on diversity rates in trials. But the impact has not been realized as expected and there are many reasons why.

227

Socioeconomic status plays a significant role in clinical trial participation. A person with a chronic disease such as cardiovascular disease, diabetes, or cancer already faces many financial demands, from medical costs to lost time at work. Additional costs for clinical trial participation can quickly become overwhelming. The cost and time spent traveling are often additional burdens in rural communities. Black and Brown people are also far less likely to participate in clinical trials. Overall, they make up 5% or fewer of clinical trial participants in cancer and cardiovascular trials. This is true even though they suffer at the same rates or higher from these diseases than do non-Latino Whites. Barriers include distrust of the healthcare system, low health literacy, lack of cultural awareness in recruitment efforts, and implicit bias or even outright racism among healthcare providers who tend to be the ones to recommend patients for a trial.

Health disparity shows its ugly head in many ways. Let's not forget that clinical trial participation is one of them.

An important result from this lack of diversity is that many guidelines will recommend a drug or a diet for all adults even when such recommendations are founded in research almost exclusively on White participants. Different races can differ in how they metabolize drugs and vitamins as well as the way metabolic disease presents and progresses. For example, it has been shown that Black individuals absorb calcium more efficiently than other ethnic groups. Criteria to diagnose metabolic syndrome differs among ethnic populations, highlighting the potential need for different metabolic health recommendations.

The American Heart Association was criticized for the "under-representation of women, elderly patients, and racial minorities in the randomized trials" used in their cardiovascular guidelines, according to a 2014 "research letter" published in the Journal of the American Medical Association.

~

I will die sooner than later, much sooner than I had ever imagined. I am 50 years old as I write. I was 45 when I was diagnosed. Most oncologists say that my dream should have been just to make it to 50. I did that. I'm at the statistical outer edge, beating the odds pretty extraordinarily.

Yay me.

My goals have changed. I used to have lots of dreams for my future. Now, they are all for other people, most prominently for my kids. I will die a lot sooner than I had ever imagined but I will be my children's mom forever.

~

Facebook
October 2, 2021

Lung cancer is the leading cause of cancer death by far. Each year, more people die of lung cancer than colon, breast, and prostate cancers combined. Ten to twenty percent of lung cancer is in patients who, like me, never smoked. Non-smoker cancer victims tend to be young, thin, and fit (i.e., the person you would least expect to get cancer). Of course, the younger part means that these patients are most likely to be in a situation like mine. Leaving behind children, nephews, nieces, and the children of close family friends.

~

Noah, Ava, Luna: Don't be afraid to confront a situation or a person, no matter what or who. Just make sure, before you do, that you can back up what you're arguing for (even if you can never agree with them). Be nice, so they're willing to engage. Then go get what you want.

Don't take anything that anyone says as gospel. (Whoops. If you really took my advice, I guess you wouldn't take my word as gospel either.) If someone says, "Here's the problem, and here's how you treat it," it's worth asking yourself, "Is it, though? I want to take a minute to really understand the problem first." Does their evaluation of the problem make sense? If it doesn't, then maybe their solution doesn't make sense. And what are the little parts and especially the hidden parts that went into making them think the way they do? Go deeper than face value.

Addressing my kids like this reminds me of the times I used to talk to physician groups. I would tell them: don't be insulting to your patients. It's not that they have an inability to understand; it's that they've never been offered the opportunity to understand, because we doctors, we the medical establishment, come into most situations presuming everyone else is stupid or at least uninterested. Personally, when I explain things to my patients, their follow-up questions are always good. Appropriate, thoughtful, on-point, often things I'd never thought of. It's great to see how appreciative they feel about being *allowed* to take more part in their own care. How we *interact* with our patients is not secondary to their care. I wish that simple, intuitive, humane idea were taught in American medical schools.

Facebook
October 2, 2021 (cont'd)

I am nesting. Not the nesting that is so joyfully done before the birth of each child. No, this nesting is different. My cancer is progressing, and each day now has a question mark. I am at the same time obsessed with making sure everything is taken care of ahead of time, yet too tired and still fighting denial to make much of a dent in what I think needs to be done. Well, okay, I still have my productive days, like the one a few days ago when I cleaned 3 junk drawers. It's incredible how much you can tell about a family from the items in these collections. But productivity is on a different scale. The old me would have had the equivalent of 60 junk drawers cleaned before 7:00 am. I miss the old me.

I am still here, thanks in part to grit and part to luck, part to privilege, all boosted by science. The grit part has helped me continue to enjoy my life. And while I have had an occasional pity party over the last four-plus years, my grief has rarely been all-consuming. It just can't be. I have three kids, a husband of over 24 years, and a busy career. Cancer just did not fit into the life I led. But recently, things have changed. I am changing.

231

Last month I was found to have innumerable new brain and lung tumors. Things are not going well. At times my weakness and pain are unbearable, and if it weren't that I can't bear to say goodbye to my children, I would probably have stopped treatment immediately. However, that brings me to the harsh question: How long should I go on?

I know the short answer: as long as possible.

But it's more complicated than that. One must weigh the damage that being a "sick mom" can inflict on an already suffering family. Even our dogs are out of sorts, so imagine what is happening with my beautiful kids. My teens fully understand the gravity of the situation. This is good, but what an awful burden to have to carry around every day. They have become hyper vigilant, and even the most minor things (cough or sneeze) can ramp up their anxiety. I can't for a second imagine this being added to the difficulties of being a teenager in this age of social media and covid. Yet there they are, maintaining their grades as a high school junior (Ava) and a college freshman (Noah). Difficult tasks in the best of circumstances. How long can they keep this up?

My beautiful baby Luna, now a tween, also understands how sick I am, but we have not assigned any timeline for my survival. Sometimes she will have an outburst over something trivial at home (typical for any kiddo that age). However, she always comes back after a few minutes to apologize. Shouldn't an eleven-year-old be able just to throw a fit and not feel guilty about it?

My kids will develop grit because of having to endure such hardships at such a young age. I am sure of that. I also believe that can increase their happiness in the long term as they really understand the "don't sweat the small things" mantra and appreciate what is in front of them in the here and now. However, it also means not having a mom like mine who will always be there for support and guidance as they get older.

~

What do I want to leave? What will be important to people once I'm gone? I feel so blessed to have had the chance to do the work I do. It's been invaluable in giving me something to focus on – yet being for the benefit of others. I think I wrote this book for several reasons but one of them, maybe the main one, is to think differently. Not to accept conventional wisdom unquestioningly.

~

Facebook
December 12, 2021

It is official. I am a cat who seems to have one more life left. It has not totally sunk in yet. The Friday after Thanksgiving, Brad and I had decided to move Christmas up to the following weekend as suggested by my physicians. I likely was not going to make it until real Christmas.

Fast forward one week to when our "Christmas" was supposed to be, and I could move around, decrease my pain meds, and feel a lot better. Since then, I have continued to feel better most days!

Miracle? Maybe.

But also a lot of self-advocating and pushiness. I am now back on the medication that helped me for the first three years, after which it lost its effectiveness. There is evidence in the literature (no big randomized clinical trials) that "rechallenging"- taking a drug one has used in the past, after a drug "holiday" – may work, at least for a bit. I doubled the dose, in the hope of getting as much as possible to the brain. And it worked! It allowed me to have the most wonderful Christmas with my family. What an amazing gift. My kids will always have that to remember.

~

And then, after one month, the drug I'd been on stopped working, again.

I welcomed the New Year with my symptoms revving up once more. Pain was difficult to control.

In February 2022 I gave my last interview, from my living room, via Zoom. It felt good to make my plea once more for changing the status quo and helping people. I summoned my energy and except for my bald head – no more wigs – I don't think anyone would realize something was wrong. But after the short interview I was exhausted and realized that my part in this mission to challenge the status quo and change lives was now over.

I have loved uncovering falsehoods and deceptions, and there's so much of it in nutrition science. But as much as I wanted to address and confront, as passionate as I was about it, I have to let it go, despite how badly I feel about that.

All these plans.

Most everyone thinks I should go into hospice as they don't want me to suffer any longer. Neither do I. It is so hard on my family. Hospice seems so reasonable, but I can't help my basic personality, which is to fight until the end.

I feel confident that I have given this all I had. That, and a lot of privilege, have helped me live almost five years since it began. For that, I have to be grateful.

I will wake up tomorrow. I will be grateful and happy that my great friends are my friends, and that our Labradoodles Ollie and Fozzie are part of our family.

I will be so grateful and happy that my wonderful mother is my mother.

I will be so grateful and happy that Brad, magnificent Brad, is my husband (our 25th anniversary is not quite around the corner!) and the greatest dad.

I will be so grateful and happy – pinch-myself happy – that my beautiful kids, Noah, Ava and Luna, are my beautiful kids.

~   ~   ~

Epilogue

by Brad Hallberg

If you have read this far, thank you. I hope you have enjoyed Sarah's story and will do us the honor of granting her a few more minutes of your time. Sarah and I were fortunate beyond words to have had the last 30 years of adventures, surviving various challenges, and raising three beautiful children. Our love for each other was unconditional and uncompromising. We were a team in every sense of the word and shared all aspects of our lives. For the nearly five years that Sarah lived with her unsurvivable diagnosis, we discussed the details in the preceding pages, revisiting our life from past decades, and sadly, talking about the future we hoped for our children and me. Although Sarah would not get to experience the milestones yet to come for our children, she hoped that the qualities they had inherited from her would serve to guide them.

Despite the trials that came with her cancer, Sarah always remained the most dedicated wife and mother. No matter what terrible news she may have received from her oncologist the week or even the day before, I always knew I could come downstairs in the morning to find her with a huge cup of hot black coffee and a smile on her face. She refused to miss a single one of our children's soccer games, even when confined to a wheelchair. And you could see this same type of selfless behavior in how she cared for her patients. As a physician, Sarah had many moments where she saw unjust, misleading, or inequitable behavior that violated a written or expected agreement between patients and healthcare providers. More often than not, she was correct, and motivated to identify the causes of the injustice and work to solve the problem. Sarah was relentless, tireless, and always searching for a way to improve the lives of those she cared about.

Sarah always had the qualities of the person you see in her TEDx talk, or listened to in her last podcast interview with Dr. Peter Attia. She was always that person...she just needed to trust her instincts and the intentions of others to set herself free. The Sarah you see in the interview with Dr. Attia is the Sarah I knew from the very beginning. Kind, genuine, thoughtful, forward-thinking, and full of passion. Sarah was intelligent, ferociously caring, and a tremendous listener of words and observer of tone, body language, circumstances, and intent. Sarah was passionate.

From 2009 until her passing, Sarah was fulfilled with her family and career. Her life became one of paying it forward and helping others. To paraphrase entrepreneur Naval Ravikant, Sarah's life was guided by "not thinking *of* herself, but thinking *for* herself, not thinking *for* others, but thinking *of* others." By being active in the world, experiencing everything it had to offer, the best parts of Sarah came to be. She believed there was something to learn from everyone, and she grew and became her best self by loving, listening, getting to know and helping people. Acting as a champion for her patients made Sarah "Dr. Sarah."

In the last four and a half years of our marriage we grew closer than ever. In that time, we realized what truly mattered. We shared everything...*everything*. We were lovingly kind, peaceful, and caring towards one another. We had only one argument during this time: It was in late January of 2022 and Sarah wanted to try one last round of chemo. Her amazing oncology and palliative care team tried to dissuade her as the risks far outweighed the benefits. I felt like I had to speak up because our daughter's first high school prom was in April. Sarah desperately wanted to see Ava, our older daughter, in the dress they had picked out together. Like most arguments over the course of our marriage, Sarah won. However, her body and mind could not handle the brutal side effects of two rounds of chemo, and sadly, she entered hospice two days after the second round.

We converted the front room of our home into a bedroom for Sarah and, with our hospice team, made it as comfortable as possible. Sarah and I slept each night by our fireplace with our two Australian Labradoodles at the end of her bed. She loved these pups and considered them the grandchildren she would otherwise never have. Slowly and inevitably, she worsened, and each day that Noah, Ava, and Luna were not in school they spent hours sitting with or lying next to their mom, holding her hand, talking about all of the great memories and how much they loved each other.

During her final week, Sarah regressed to the point where she no longer had the strength to speak. She could hear us, hold hands, blink, cry, and show us how much she loved each of us. At this time, I decided that the kids should each have a moment with their mom that might end up being the last words their mother would ever hear from them. Noah, Ava, and Luna took as much time as needed to share their private thoughts with their mother. When Luna, who had recently turned 12 years old, went to see her mom, I was worried she might have trouble and stayed close. I heard Luna say to her mother, "Mom, I love you. I love you and I know you love us with everything you've got. You did your best. You did your best, mom! You need to know you are the best mom! . . . and, it's okay for you to go. It's okay for you to rest. Everything will be okay. We love you, and we will be okay." Sarah understood everything Luna was saying as I heard her cry, trembling with so much emotion the bed rails rattled. Sarah felt the way only a mother could while listening to her daughter say these words. Listening to Luna and Sarah was brutally difficult for me, the most heartbreaking moment. Luna spoke to her mom with such courage, passion, and strength. Strength that I did not realize she had within her young heart . . . but I'm sure Sarah knew.

During our final evenings in hospice, I occasionally gave Sarah a dose of Haldol, a powerful anti-psychotic that calms patients quickly when most other things are not effective. Early in the morning on March 28th, 2022, I woke up next to Sarah and heard her speaking calmly and more clearly than at any time over the previous two weeks. At first I thought she was going to become agitated and was considering preparing a dose of Haldol. But her agitation never materialized and I did not have to administer the antipsychotic. Instead of agitation, her rate of breathing slowed and she became very calm, which I didn't expect. I sat there listening to her breathing and held her hand. For nearly an hour she was so peaceful. Then something happened that I was prepared for but not expecting. While I held her hand, her breathing stopped, and Sarah was finally able to rest.

Sarah had a few basic principles she lived by and asked me to share them with you: love your family and friends, never stop learning, be kind, advocate for yourself and your children, seek the truth, travel, and always do your best!!

I wish everyone could have known Sarah the way I did. She was truly amazing.

Sarah, until I see you again.

Love, your #1 fan ☺

Acknowledgments

Like all innovators and activists, Sarah stood on the shoulders of – and held hands with – many others.

First, thank you to Sarah's patients and trial participants. She loved each and every one. She understood the often-difficult commitment they were making. They helped keep her going through fatigue and then illness.

"Thank you" can't begin to say it all to Tamara Hazbun, Sarah's close friend and colleague, the person with whom just hours before her seizure she had shared the joy of her "perfect" life. The times Tamara came to the hospital and the house to visit and comfort when Sarah was going through one of the many (really) bad times are too numerous to count.

Andrew Postman has been patient, understanding, and dedicated, a true professional during the development of Sarah's story. His ability to turn her raw thoughts into a powerful and engaging narrative is impressive. It has been no easy feat to genuinely capture Sarah's assertive voice.

Sarah received so much emotional support and practical help from so many friends, including the Strachans, the Gramas, the Mumfords, Warren Ng, and Erika Ugianskis.

Thanks to the amazing staff at IU Health Arnett Medical Weight Loss Clinic, whose enthusiasm and energy made its many successes possible: Joni

Anderson, MA; Amanda Dehne, RN; Monica Keyes, NP; Patti McKee, MA; Zachary Roberts, MA; and Danielle Wharff, RN.

The Virta team always did what it took, including, in some cases, moving to Lafayette, Indiana. They were all extraordinarily supportive: Sami Inkinen; Dr. Shaminie Athinarayanan; Dr. Jim McCarter; Dr. Amy McKenzie; and Dr. Brittanie Volk.

Thank you to the often-unsung heroes of any study project, the logistics experts: Rachael Bolden, Sydney Rivera, and Deklin Veenhuizen.

Thanks so much to the health coaches, including Brent Creighton, Marcy Abner, Bobbie Glon, and Theresa Link.

For their pioneering research and writing, which inspired and motivated Sarah, appreciation and gratitude to Dr. Stephen Phinney, Dr. Jeff Volek, and Dr. Eric Westman. Kudos to the science journalists who persevere in getting the word out to the public about the benefits of carbohydrate restriction, despite vociferous and often vitriolic pushback – especially Nina Teicholz and Gary Taubes.

Thanks to all those who provided valuable insights and substantive contributions to the book, including Dr. Saleh Aldasouqi, Senator Bob Kerrey, and Dr. Jennifer Trilk. Thank you to Robert Walsh for his careful reading and suggestions.

Hugs to Dr. Dale Brown, Professor of Exercise Physiology at Illinois State University, who helped inspire Sarah to follow her professional path. Unlike many others, he let Sarah be Sarah as she energized all over the place. He also introduced her to research. Little did either of them know what that would lead to.

Glossary

Sarah knew that lots of medical terms were so common doctors often assumed everyone had the same understanding. She was insistent that everyone understand these terms (though some do get, as she would say, "kind of wonky").

A1c
Hemoglobin A1c or HbA1c, commonly stated simply as A1c. It measures blood sugar levels, as a percentage, and is the common indicator of diabetes or prediabetes. The levels are:

Normal A1c is under 5.7% without medication.

Prediabetes is 5.7% to 6.4% or less than 6.5% with metformin.

Diabetes is equal to or greater than 6.5% or less than 6.5% with diabetes medication other than metformin.

Blood Sugar (Blood Glucose)
A result of the breakdown (metabolism) of the food we consume, especially from carbohydrates. The blood carries sugar to the body's cells where it is used to produce energy. Insulin, produced by the pancreas, is the "key" that unlocks the cells for the sugar to enter. See **Diabetes** for detail.

Carbohydrates (Carbs)

One of the three components of nutrition – carbohydrates, fats, and proteins. They provide the calories needed for energy plus materials needed for growth and repair.

Carbohydrates come in various forms, including starches and simple sugars. Foods high in carbohydrates include wheat flour (so . . . bread, cake, cookies, crackers, pretzels, pizza crust, tortillas, etc.), rice and other grains (such as oats, corn, barley, farro), potatoes, sugar you add in cooking and at the table, plus the many processed foods containing sugar.

Note that the sugars in processed foods are often disguised using names like corn sweetener, corn syrup, or cane syrup. Honey, molasses, and maple syrups are also essentially pure sugar.

Carbohydrates are also present at high levels in most fruits and fruit juices and some vegetables, especially root veggies (think sweet potatoes, carrots, beets), peas, and legumes (dried beans). Fresh milk (whether full-fat or skim) also contains a sugar called lactose. One quart of milk contains as many carbs as three slices of bread.

Carbohydrate Intolerance

The body's insulin production cannot handle the level of blood sugar produced by the breakdown of carbohydrates. In effect, carbohydrate consumption is too high. The body can't tolerate that level. "That level" varies among individuals. See **Diabetes** for detail.

Cardiovascular Disease

Diseases of the heart and blood vessels. Risk factors include low HDL-C, high triglycerides, high triglyceride/HDL ratio, diabetes, obesity, and high blood pressure.

Control Group

In clinical research studies (trials), participants are usually divided into two groups. Individuals in the control group do not receive the treatment or intervention that is the basis of the study. In our study, members of the control group did not participate in the very low-carb (ketogenic) diet or have health coaches. They continued with the standard of care for diabetes – consultation with their doctors and standard diabetes education. See **Experimental Group**.

Diabetes

When you eat carbohydrates, your body breaks them down to a simple sugar called blood glucose, (or just glucose), commonly called blood sugar (or just sugar). As the name indicates, whether from digested foods or body stores, this sugar enters your blood and is carried to the cells of your body. In response to the rise in blood sugar, your pancreas releases the hormone insulin which allows cells to absorb the sugar. I like to refer to insulin as the key that unlocks the cells so they can receive the sugar. Doing so reduces the level of sugar in the blood – something we want. The sugar that goes into your cells is used for energy.

Basically, diabetes is a disease manifested by elevated blood sugar. It is typically diagnosed if you have fasting blood sugar above 126 mg/dl or a blood A1c at or above 6.5%.

For medical purposes, diabetes is classified in two forms – type 1 and type 2. NOTE that I am talking only about type 2 diabetes where in most cases the pancreas can still make insulin. With type 1 diabetes, the pancreas produces little or no insulin. The cause of type 1 diabetes is typically an autoimmune disorder in which the immune system mistakenly attacks insulin-producing cells. So if you have type 1 diabetes, your insulin dose may be reduced on a low-carb diet, but you will still need to take insulin.

For the last five decades, type 2 diabetes has been thought of as a disease of insulin resistance. The level of insulin resistance varies from individual to individual. The cause is not fully known, but genetics is part of it. That's why family history is important in evaluating the risk for diabetes.

For individuals with insulin resistance, insulin production cannot handle the level of blood sugar produced by the breakdown of carbohydrates. The key does not fit so the doors to the cells won't open and sugar in the blood cannot be absorbed by the cells as rapidly as necessary. As a result the body makes more keys and the system is flooded with insulin. For someone with IR, the pancreas will keep on producing the higher levels of insulin . . . until it can't. Over time, and this can be years, the insulin-making cells die from overuse, insulin production goes down, and blood sugar rises. This is type 2 diabetes. Now the body has to be coaxed into producing more insulin – with medication – and if that doesn't work, insulin has to be added – by injection or by pump.

A newer approach to type 2 diabetes is to view it as a disease of carbohydrate intolerance. It is variable among individuals. In this context, type 2 diabetes can be thought of as a kind of food intolerance, meaning your body cannot deal with the rise in blood sugar caused by consuming carbohydrates above your threshold. Think about other food intolerances, such as lactose or gluten.

Insulin resistance and carbohydrate intolerance can be seen as two sides of the same coin. Both describe the same eventual scenario – carbohydrate intake becomes too high for an individual's insulin production to handle. And here's the hook: A diagnosis of insulin resistance "calls for" drugs to reduce the resistance or to deliver more insulin – the current standard medical approach. But given a diagnosis of carbohydrate intolerance, the natural thing to do is to cut carbs down to the point that the body can manage them. You don't recommend that a person with lactose intolerance drink more milk; why would you recommend that someone with a carbohydrate intolerance eat more carbs, or continue following a high carb diet? Insulin resistance and carbohydrate intolerance – the same coin, but you come to different treatment reactions depending which side is up.

Since the use of insulin in the 1920s, medical practitioners have usually seen – been taught to see – the insulin resistance side of the coin. No doubt about it, insulin is a miracle drug for people with type 1 diabetes, whose bodies produce little or no insulin and for those whose pancreas (the insulin-producing organ) has been damaged or removed. But for the vast majority of diabetes patients who have type 2, the insulin approach is often damaging. For instance, insulin is a fat storage hormone. When the pancreas is producing extra insulin to deal with the excess sugar in your blood, your body goes on storage mode for fat. The excess blood sugar is stored in the liver and fat cells, which convert it to fat.

And here's something else to consider: A carb is a carb. So once you consume to your tolerance level, even healthy carbs will be more than your cells can absorb for energy and there will be an insulin surge. Carbohydrates are considered healthy if they are unprocessed whole foods rich in fiber and nutrients. These are the kinds of carbs we encourage but the limits still apply.

If you continuously consume above your carbohydrate tolerance, your pancreas produces more and more insulin to try to remove the sugar from your blood. That fat storage hormone is around all the time at elevated levels, which means that fat deposited in your fat cells has a hard time coming back out to be burned for energy.

Not everyone who is obese has diabetes and not everyone with diabetes is overweight – but you can see why there is so much connection.

Diabetes Reversal
A1c goes, and stays, below 6.5 without insulin or other medications (except sometimes metformin). Diabetes reversal is a goal of the very low-carbohydrate (ketogenic) diet.

Experimental Group
In clinical research studies (trials), participants are basically divided into two groups. Individuals in the experimental group, sometimes called the intervention

or the treatment group, receive the "treatment" that is the basis of the study. Examples in health studies are a drug, a vaccine, a medical device. In our study the treatment was the low-carb diet and the use of health coaches. See **Control Group.**

Glucose
See **Blood Sugar**.

HDL-C (High-Density Lipoprotein)
Often known as the "good" cholesterol because it carries cholesterol to the liver where it is eliminated from the body. HDL over 40 mgl/dL in men and over 50 mg/dL in women are the benchmarks for healthy HDL levels. Low HDL is one of the markers for metabolic syndrome.

Health Coach
In our trial and at Virta, a health coach is a trained consultant who is in contact with patients via monitors and apps, also text and sometimes video. The coach receives messages from the monitors (e.g., a patient's blood sugar level) and can contact the patient essentially in real time with questions and advice. In consultation with the patient's physician, medications can be altered, as can carbohydrate restriction (up or down). The coaches also encourage and congratulate. The patient can contact the coach with questions or for advice. We say it's like having a physician and a health counselor in your pocket. Personal, individualized therapy by health coaches contributes to patient success on a low carbohydrate or ketogenic diet and to sustainability.

Insulin

A hormone that is released from the pancreas in response to rising blood sugar. Insulin pushes blood sugar into cells where it is used for energy. When used as a drug, insulin is given by injection or pump. See **Diabetes** for detail.

Insulin Resistance

Insulin is the "key" to open muscle and other cells to let in blood sugar, which is then used for energy. If the cells do not respond normally – resist using the insulin – the pancreas keeps producing more. The extra production of insulin will keep blood sugar seemingly under control for a time, but eventually insulin production will not be sufficient and blood sugar will rise to prediabetes levels and then to type 2 diabetes. See **Diabetes** for detail.

Ketogenic (Keto) Diet

The ketogenic diet, commonly known as "keto" has become popular enough in recent years that it has taken on a life of its own, a life that can be complicated and confusing with varying definitions and recommendations in the popular press, from social media influencers, and in advertising.

A ketogenic diet is a very low-carbohydrate diet. In our clinic we talk about "a well-formulated" ketogenic diet. By that, we mean nutritionally well formulated (no, it's not just meat and cheese) and that it is not one size fits all. Although we usually start our patients on a maximum of 30 grams of carbs a day, it really depends on the individual's metabolic health. So some individuals with diabetes or other indicators of poor metabolic health may start with under 20 carbs a day. For others, the upper limit can be 50 grams. As a percentage of calories, 5-10% are carbs, 15-20% is protein, and 70-80% is fat.

The focus of the ketogenic diet is twofold: replacing most carbohydrates with fats – including saturated fats (but not trans fats) – and keeping protein at a moderate level. Protein intake is individualized depending on one's biomarkers, but generally aims at 1.5 grams per kg of ideal body weight.

The goal is to increase your body's production of ketones, which are compounds that form during the metabolism of fat from your food or the fat stored in your body. The presence of ketones (a state known as ketosis) is evidence that your body is now primarily using fat, not carbohydrates, as its main energy source. In effect, when the body isn't driven to burn lots of carbs, blood insulin levels fall, and your body is given "permission" to use fat – lots of it! Of course, when stored fat is used, you will lose weight, even when you eat each meal until you are full.

The ketone level is easily measured from a drop of blood, taken by pricking the finger, the same way you might monitor blood sugar. Other measures using urine or breath testing are much less accurate and often cause more confusion than help.

A misconception about the ketogenic diet is that these individuals will always be this carb-restricted. And frankly, for some individuals that will be true if they want to stay healthy. But many people will be able to adjust their carb consumption upward to some extent, after they have achieved their desirable weight loss and kept their type 2 diabetes at bay for months or a few years. Of course they cannot go back to their old typical American pattern of 300-400 grams of carbohydrates a day if they want to maintain their diabetes reversal, or stay out of prediabetes, or maintain their weight loss. I want to emphasize: carbohydrate restriction does not cure diabetes. It is a reversal and that reversal can be maintained only with an adequate and personalized degree of carb restriction. For most folks starting out with diabetes that will probably mean a maximum of 50 grams a day, although some people may explore a somewhat higher level and remain in type 2 diabetes reversal.

Ketones (Ketone bodies)
Produced by the breakdown of fats and used as fuel by the body, instead of blood sugar, if carbohydrate consumption has been restricted.

Ketosis
In ketosis, the body's primary source of energy is fat and ketones, not blood sugar. Ketones are produced when the body breaks down fat – consumed or stored – instead of carbohydrates. After adopting a very low carb diet it can take several days to a week or more to be "in ketosis." To stay in ketosis, the restriction on carbohydrate intake will vary among individuals, but will usually be around 50 grams a day.

Low-Carbohydrate Diet
Low-carb is generally defined as allowing a maximum of 25% of calories as carbohydrates, or less than 130 grams a day.

LDL (or LDL-C: Low-density lipoprotein cholesterol)

(The -C stands for calculated. It is not a direct measure.) Often known as the "bad" cholesterol because high levels were thought to increase the risk for cardiovascular disease. For most individuals on a very low-carb (ketogenic) diet LDL-C does not change.

A subset of people on a ketogenic diet will experience an increase in their LDL-C. We have no long-term data on this phenomenon and its health risks, if any. For some people, LDL goes up with weight loss and comes back down again when weight stabilizes. For those for whom LDL-C stays up, though, Virta physicians continue to prescribe statins to be on the safe side. We will need additional research to determine how much to use statins, if at all. Note that on a low-carb diet, HDL typically goes up (good) and triglycerides drop dramatically (very good) and there is vast improvement in the triglycerides/HDL ratio, an important cardiovascular risk factor.

Using the NMR blood test, a direct measure of cholesterol, we also look at LDL-P (the "P" stands for particles and is a count of the total number of LDL particles in circulation). The NMR is not routinely ordered but LDL-P is a better indicator of cardiovascular risk than the standard measures. In patients on low-carb and ketogenic diets, we often see an increase in the large, buoyant LDL particles (good LDL) and a decrease in the small, dense particles (bad LDL). Low carb is a potent stimulus to reduce those small particles for most people.

Macronutrients
The primary components of nutrition — carbohydrates, fats, and proteins. They provide the calories needed for energy, plus materials needed for growth and repair. They are usually measured in grams.

Metabolic Disease
A broad umbrella designation for what is now thought to be the basis of many chronic diseases, including type 2 diabetes, prediabetes, metabolic syndrome, cardiovascular disease, some cancers, even Alzheimer's, and depression. Although the most prevalent metabolic disease is overweight/obesity, people who are not overweight can have other metabolic diseases.

Metabolic Syndrome
A clinical assessment (medical diagnosis) of biomarkers for disease risk, especially type 2 diabetes and cardiovascular risk. The markers are:

high blood pressure: more than 120/80 mg/dl or use of hypertension medication. Some practitioners use 140 or 130 for the systolic (upper) measure

high triglycerides: more that 150 mg/dL (some practitioners use more than 100)

waist circumference (truncal obesity – the famous apple shape): a waist circumference over 35 inches for women, over 40 inches for men (for people of Southeast Asian, Chinese or Japanese descent, it's 35.5 inches for men and 31.5 inches for women)

elevated blood sugar: A1c over 6.5% (5.7% to 6.4% is prediabetes)

low HDL-C: under 50 mg/dL for women, under 40 mg/dL for men

A diagnosis of three of these markers is considered metabolic syndrome. Any one of these bio-markers indicates risk for cardiovascular disease and type 2 diabetes. But the sum of these parts is more than the individual pieces. In other words, the presence of multiple risk markers means the risk of heart disease or diabetes increases considerably.

Metabolism

Complex chemical processes within our bodies that, at base, keep us alive and functioning. It includes how food – which provides the necessary macro and micronutrients – is broken down and converted into energy. "Energy" is more than physical movement and includes everything your body does – growing, cell maintenance and repair, breathing, etc. For our purposes, we use metabolism to mean this breakdown of food.

Micronutrients

Do not provide calories but are required for the body to function. Think vitamins and minerals. They are usually measured in small units, milligrams or micrograms.

Obesity

A body mass index (BMI) of 30 and over. A BMI of 25-30 is considered overweight. You can calculate your BMI: Square your height in inches; divide your weight in pounds by your squared height; multiply by 703. Example: weight = 148 pounds, height = 64 inches (5'4")

64x64 = 4096
148/4096 x 703 = 25.4

Or you can go online and search for a BMI Calculator

The CDC estimates that 42% of Americans are obese and 32% are overweight. That's almost three-quarters of us!

Prediabetes

Prediabetes is a description of the behavior of blood sugar before actual diabetes. It describes an earlier stage of insulin resistance where blood sugar is elevated above normal, but not high enough to be called type 2 diabetes.

Normal A1c is under 5.7% without medication.

Prediabetes is 5.7% to 6.4% or 6.5% with metformin.

Diabetes is equal to or greater than 6.5% or less than 6.5% with diabetes medication other than metformin.

Pre-prediabetes

Pre-prediabetes is not often discussed or described, but paying more attention to it could help prevent the occurrence of prediabetes and then full-blown diabetes. Markers such as A1c might be in the normal range, but beneath those normal markers the body is working extra hard to maintain them, especially blood sugar level. Insulin levels may already be elevated as may blood sugar levels in the two hours after a meal.

Saturated Fat
A type of fat that has in the past been identified as an unhealthy fat, especially as a cardiovascular risk factor and as responsible for weight gain. Recent research – such as our trial – has shown that carbohydrates are more responsible. We showed that an increase in fat, including saturated fat, and a decrease in carbohydrates, reduce cardiovascular risk and can result in considerable weight loss. Saturated fats include most animal fats, whole fat dairy products, and coconut and palm kernel oils.

Sugar
See **Blood Sugar**.

Triglycerides
A kind of fat in the blood and stored as body fat until needed for energy, like between meals. A healthy triglyceride level is considered to under 150 mg/dl, although some practitioners use 100 mg/dl. High triglycerides are a cardiovascular risk and one of the markers for metabolic syndrome.

Waist Circumference
Sometimes called truncal obesity (the famous apple shape): a waist circumference over 35 inches for women, over 40 inches for men (for people of Southeast Asian, Chinese or Japanese descent, it's 35.5 inches for men and 31.5 inches for women). Truncal obesity is a marker for metabolic syndrome and suggests what has been called pre-prediabetes.

Going Public

On top of her many scientific publications (see next section), Sarah wrote (or in the case of *The New York Times* article, co-wrote with Dr. Osama Hamdy) for mainstream publications as well, because she knew how important it was to get the word out to the general public:

- "Before You Spend $26,000 on Weight-Loss Surgery, Do This,"[52] *The New York Times*, September 10, 2016
- "Don't manage diabetes, reverse it,"[53] *The Detroit News*, June 5, 2018
- "Government Dietary Guidelines Are Plain Wrong: Avoid Carbs, Not Fat,"[54] *The Hill,* November 29, 2018
- "I'm a doctor with Stage 4 cancer during a pandemic,"[55] *Tampa Bay Times*, July 5, 2020

---

[52] nytimes.com/2016/09/11/opinion/sunday/before-you-spend-26000-on-weight-loss-surgery-do-this.html

[53] detroitnews.com/story/opinion/2018/06/05/opinion-dont-manage-diabetes-reverse/670756002/

[54] thehill.com/opinion/healthcare/419020-government-dietary-guidelines-are-plain-wrong-avoid-carbs-not-fat

[55] tampabay.com/opinion/2020/07/05/im-a-doctor-with-stage-4-cancer-during-a-pandemic-column/

Peer-Reviewed, Published Papers

from the Virta-IUH Trial

1. Lyman KS, Athinarayanan SJ, McKenzie AL, Pearson CL, Adams RN, Hallberg SJ, McCarter JP, Volek JS, Phinney SD, Andrawis JP. "Continuous Care Intervention with Carbohydrate Restriction Improves Physical Function of the Knees among Patients with Type 2 Diabetes: A Non-randomized Study." *BMC Musculoskeletal Disorders.* 2022 Mar; 23(1):297. pubmed.ncbi.nlm.nih.gov/35351093/

2. Adams RN, Athinarayanan SJ, McKenzie AL, Hallberg SJ, McCarter JP, Phinney SD, Gonzalez JS. "Depressive Symptoms Improve over 2 Years of Type 2 Diabetes Treatment via a Digital Continuous Remote Care Intervention Focused on Carbohydrate Restriction." *J Behav Med.* 2022 Jun; 45(3):416-427. pubmed.ncbi.nlm.nih.gov/35084637/

3. McKenzie AL, Athinarayanan SJ, McCue J, Adams RN, Keyes M, McCarter JP, Volek JS, Phinney SD, Hallberg SJ. "Type 2 Diabetes Prevention Focused on Normalization of Glycemia." *Nutrients* 2021 Mar; 13(3):749. ncbi.nlm.nih.gov/pmc/articles/PMC7996820/

4. Athinarayanan SJ, Hallberg SJ, McKenzie AL, Lechner K, King S, McCarter JP, Volek JS, Phinney SD, Krauss RM. "Impact of a 2-Year Trial of Nutritional Ketosis on Indices of Cardiovascular Disease Risk in Patients with Type 2 Diabetes." *Cardiovasc Diabetol.* 2020 dEC; 19(1):208. pubmed.ncbi.nlm.nih.gov/33292205/

5. Hallberg SJ, Dockter NE, Kushner JA, Athinarayanan SJ. "Improving the Scientific Rigour of Nutritional Recommendations for Adults with Type 2 Diabetes: A Comprehensive Review of the American Diabetes Association Guideline-Recommended Eating Patterns." *Diabetes Obes Metab.* 2019 Aug; 21(8):1769-1779. dom-pubs.pericles-prod.literatumonline.com/doi/10.1111/dom.13736

6. Hallberg SJ, Gershuni VM, Hazbun TL, Athinarayanan SJ. "Reversing Type 2 Diabetes: A Narrative Review of the Evidence." *Nutrients* 2019 Apr 1; 11(4):766. pubmed.ncbi.nlm.nih.gov/30939855/

7. Athinarayanan SJ, Adams RN, Hallberg SJ, McKenzie AL, Bhanpuri NH, Campbell WW, Volek JS, Phinney SD, McCarter JP. "Long-Term Effects of a Novel Continuous Remote Care Intervention Including Nutritional Ketosis for the Management of Type 2 Diabetes: A 2-year Non-randomized Clinical Trial." *Frontiers in Endocrinology* 2019 Jun; 10:348.

pubmed.ncbi.nlm.nih.gov/31231311/

8. Vilar-Gomez E, Athinarayanan SJ, Adams RN, Hallberg SJ, Bhanpuri NH, McKenzie AL, Campbell WW, McCarter JP, Phinney SD, Volek JS, Chalasani N. "Post Hoc Analyses of Surrogate Markers of Non-alcoholic Fatty Liver Disease (NAFLD) and Liver Fibrosis in Patients with Type 2 Diabetes in a Digitally Supported Continuous Care Intervention: An Open-Label, Non-Randomised Controlled Study." *BMJ Open.* 2019 Feb; 9:e023597. pubmed.ncbi.nlm.nih.gov/30803948/

9. Siegmann MS, Athinarayanan SJ, Hallberg SJ, McKenzie AL, Bhanpuri NH, Campbell WW, McCarter JP, Phinney SD, Volek JS, Van Dort CJ. "Improvement in Patient-Reported Sleep in Type 2 Diabetes and Prediabetes Participants Receiving a Continuous Care Intervention with Nutritional Ketosis." *Sleep Medicine* 2019 Mar; 55:92-99. sciencedirect.com/science/article/pii/S138994 5718304945

10. Bhanpuri NH, Hallberg SJ., Williams PT, McKenzie AL, Ballard KD, Campbell WW, McCarter JP, Phinney SD, Volek JS. "Cardiovascular Disease Risk Factor Responses to a Type 2 Diabetes Care Model Including Nutritional Ketosis Induced by Sustained Carbohydrate Restriction at One Year: An Open Label, Non-Randomized, Controlled Study." *Cardiovascular Diabetology* 2018 May; 17(1):56. pubmed.ncbi.nlm.nih.gov/29712560/

11. Hallberg SJ, McKenzie AL, Williams PT, Bhanpuri NH, Peters AL, Campbell WW, Hazbun TL, Volk BM, McCarter JP, Phinney SD, Volek JS. "Effectiveness and Safety of a Novel Care Model for the Management of Type 2 Diabetes at 1 Year: An Open-Label, Non-Randomized, Controlled Study." *Diabetes Therapy* 2018 Apr; 9(2):583-612. pubmed.ncbi.nlm.nih.gov/29417495/

12. McKenzie AL, Hallberg SJ, Creighton "A Novel Intervention Including Individualized Nutritional Recommendations Reduces HbA1c, Medication Use, and Weight in Type-2 Diabetes." *JMIR Diabetes* 2017 Mar; 2(1):e5. pubmed.ncbi.nlm.nih.gov/30291062/

Suggested Reading

Sarah was often asked for book recommendations. Here's her low-carb/high-fat shortlist. These were found on her bedside table more than once.

The Art and Science of Low Carbohydrate Living: An Expert Guide to Making the Life-Saving Benefits of Carbohydrate Restriction Sustainable and Enjoyable
by Jeff S. Volek and Stephen D. Phinney
Teaches doctors about the science and implementation of a low-carb diet. However, anyone who really wants to know the details should read this book.

The Big Fat Surprise: Why Butter, Meat and Cheese Belong in a Healthy Diet by Nina Teicholz
A well-researched book about the misguided advice to avoid fat.

Why We Get Fat: And What to Do About It
by Gary Taubes
A great intro book. Explores the background and presents the science in a well-researched but easy-to-understand manner. This is the book the clinic gave to all new patients.

Good Calories, Bad Calories: Fats, Carbs, and the Controversial Science of Diet and Health by Gary Taubes

A research masterpiece for the serious fact-seeker. A very detailed history and science of carbs.

The Art and Science of Low Carbohydrate Performance by Jeff S. Volek and Stephen D. Phinney
For Athletes, Phinney and Volek's "companion" book to The Art and Science of Low Carbohydrate Living. It describes the benefits of fat-fueled energy for training, performance, and recovery.

The Low Carb Dietitian's Guide to Health and Beauty: How a Whole-Foods, Low-Carbohydrate Lifestyle Can Help You Look and Feel Better Than Ever by Franziska Spritzler
A new entry with good advice for low-carb living. More for people who wish to stay above the level for ketosis.

Endnotes

Preface

at a meeting of the American Diabetes Association: Virta Health. "Virta Health Highlights Lasting, Transformative Health Improvements In 5-Year Diabetes Reversal Study." June 5, 2022. virtahealth.com/blog/virta-sustainable-health-improvements-5-year-diabetes-reversal-study

exclusively on cardiovascular outcomes: That study, called PREDIMED and published in the *New England Journal of Medicine*, was retracted. Its findings were reissued, yet there are lingering questions about their validity, as described in this article: Agarwal A, Ioannidis PA. "PREDIMED Trial of Mediterranean Diet: Retracted, Republished, Still Trusted?" *BMJ* 2019; 364:l341. bmj.com/content/364/bmj.l341

Chapter 4: Fed Up

are more likely to die: Fenton JJ, Jerant AF, Bertakis KD, Franks P. "The Cost of Satisfaction: A National Study of Patient Satisfaction, Health Care Utilization, Expenditures, and Mortality." *Arch Intern Med.* 2012; 172(5):405-411.

jamanetwork.com/journals/jamainternalmedicine/fullar
ticle/1108766

Chapter 5: Rock My World

any more than low-fat dairy: O'Sullivan TA, Schmidt KA, Kratz M. "Whole-Fat or Reduced-Fat Dairy Product Intake, Adiposity, and Cardiometabolic Health in Children: A Systematic Review." *Advances in Nutrition* 2020 Jul; 11(4):928-950.
pubmed.ncbi.nlm.nih.gov/32119732/

likely to lead to childhood obesity: Beck AL, Heyman M, Chao C, Wojcicki J. "Full Fat Milk Consumption Protects against Severe Childhood Obesity in Latinos." *Preventive Medicine Reports* 2017 Dec; 8:1-5.
doi.org/10.1016/j.pmedr.2017.07.005

began to issue the Guidelines: "History of the Dietary Guidelines." Dietary Guidelines for Americans.
dietaryguidelines.gov/about-dietary-guidelines/history-dietary-guidelines

promote health, and prevent disease: U.S. Department of Health and Human Services. Office of Disease Prevention and Health Promotion. "Dietary Guidelines for Americans."
health.gov/our-work/nutrition-physical-activity/dietary-guidelines/current-dietary-guidelines

the current body of nutrition science: U.S. Department of Health and Human Services. Office of Disease

Prevention and Health Promotion. "Dietary Guidelines for Americans."
health.gov/our-work/nutrition-physical-activity/dietary-guidelines

versus low-fat have been ignored: Wharton J. "Blog: USDA Excluding Virtually all Low-Carb Studies." *Low-Carb Action Network* May 13, 2020. lowcarbaction.org/usda-continues-to-exclude-low-carb-studies/

yogurt, and cheese, and lean meats: U.S. Department of Agriculture and U.S. Department of Health and Human Services. *Dietary Guidelines for Americans, 2020-2025*. 9th Edition. December 2020. dietaryguidelines.gov/resources/2020-2025-dietary-guidelines-online-materials

Chapter 7: It's Not the Patient's Fault

keep from regaining still more: Anekwe C. "Exercise, Metabolism, and Weight: New Research from *The Biggest Loser*." *Harvard Health Publishing* January 27, 2022. health.harvard.edu/blog/exercise-metabolism-and-weight-new-research-from-the-biggest-loser-202201272676

Chapter 8: Rock My World, Again

exercise is not a good plan to lose weight: Cox CE. "Role of Physical Activity for Weight Loss and Weight Maintenance." *Diabetes Spectrum* 2017 Aug; 30(3):157–160.
doi.org/10.2337/ds17-0013

Chapter 9: What IS Going On?

fat consumption was far weaker: Yerushalmy J, Hilleboe HE. "Fat in the Diet and Mortality from Heart Disease: A Methodologic Note." *New York State Journal of Medicine* 1957 Jul; 57(14):2343-54.
thescienceofnutrition.files.wordpress.com/2014/03/fat-in-the-diet-and-mortality-from-heart-disease1.pdf

in a special publication by the American Heart Association (AHA): *Circulation* April 1, 1970 - Volume 41, Issue 4s1.

correlated strongly with heart disease deaths: Menotti A, Kromhout D, Blackburn H, Fidanza F, Buzina R, Nissinen A. For the Seven Countries Study Research Group. "Food Intake Patterns and 25-Year Mortality from Coronary Heart Disease: Cross-Cultural Correlations in the Seven Countries Study. The Seven Countries Study Research Group." *European Journal of Epidemiology* 1999 Jul; 15(6):507-15.
pubmed.ncbi.nlm.nih.gov/10485342/

decreased saturated fat in the blood!: Astrup A, Magkos F, Bier DM, Brenna JT, de Oliveira Otto MC, Hill JO, King JC, Mente A, Ordovas JM, Volek JS, Yusuf S, Krauss RM. "Saturated Fats and Health: A Reassessment and Proposal for Food-Based Recommendations: JACC State-of-the-Art Review." *Journal of the American College of Cardiology* 2020 Aug; 76(7): 844-857. doi.org/10.1016/j.jacc.2020.05.077

Forsythe CE, Phinney SD, Fernandez ML, Quann EE, Wood RJ, Bibus DM, Kraemer WJ, Feinman RD, Volek JS. "Comparison of Low-Fat and Low Carbohydrate Diets on Circulating Fatty Acid Composition and Markers of Inflammation." *Lipids* 2008 Jan; 43(1):65-77. pubmed.ncbi.nlm.nih.gov/18046594/

especially of the liver and pancreas: Giovannucci E, Harlan DM, Archer MC, Bergenstal RM, Gapstur SM, Habel LA, Pollak M, Regensteiner JG, Yee D. "Diabetes and Cancer: A Consensus Report." *Diabetes Care* 2010 Jul; 33(7):1674–1685. ncbi.nlm.nih.gov/pmc/articles/PMC2890380/

compatible with life apparently is zero…": Institute of Medicine of the National Academies; Food and Nutrition Board; Panel on Macronutrients, Panel on the Definition of Dietary Fiber, Subcommittee on Upper Reference Levels of Nutrients, Subcommittee on Interpretation and Uses of Dietary Reference Intakes, and the Standing Committee on the Scientific Evaluation of Dietary Reference Intakes."*Dietary Reference Intakes for Energy, Carbohydrate, Fiber,*

Fat, Fatty Acids, Cholesterol, Protein, and Amino Acids. Chapter 6, Dietary Carbohydrates: Sugars and Starches: 265. Washington, DC: National Academies Press. 2005.
nap.nationalacademies.org/read/10490/chapter/8

about the dangers of saturated fat: Sacks FM, Lichtenstein AH, Wu JHY, Appel LJ, Creager MA, Kris-Etherton PM, Miller M, Rimm EB, Rudel LL, Robinson JG, Stone NJ, Van Horn LV and On behalf of the American Heart Association. "Dietary Fats and Cardiovascular Disease: A Presidential Advisory from the American Heart Association." *Circulation* 2017; 136:e1–e23.
ahajournals.org/doi/full/10.1161/CIR.00000000000005 10

the Mediterranean diet study: Kris-Etherton P, Eckel RH, Howard BV, St. Jeor S, Bazzarre TL, for the Nutrition Committee Population Science Committee and Clinical Science Committee of the American Heart Association. "Lyon Diet Heart Study: Benefits of a Mediterranean-Style, National Cholesterol Education Program/American Heart Association Step I Dietary Pattern on Cardiovascular Disease." *Circulation* 2001; 103,(3):1823–1825.
ahajournals.org/doi/full/10.1161/01.cir.103.13.1823

Chapter 10: What IS Going On? Part 2

generalized and applied to the greater US population: Food4Health Alliance. "Limitations of the Evidence on

Race, Ethnicity, and Socio-economic Status in the Report by the 2020 Dietary Guidelines Advisory Committee." August 2020. food4health.org/wp-content/uploads/2020/08/F4H-report-113p.pdf

almost guaranteed to attract little notice: Frantz Jr. ID, Dawson EA, Ashman PL, Gatewood LC, Bartsch GE, Kuba K, Brewer ER. "Test of Effect of Lipid Lowering by Diet on Cardiovascular Risk: The Minnesota Coronary Survey." *Arteriosclerosis: An Official Journal of the American Heart Association, Inc.* 1989 Jan; 9(1):129-135. ahajournals.org/doi/epdf/10.1161/01.ATV.9.1.129

die of a heart attack: Ramsden CE, Zamora D, Majchrzak-Hong S, Faurot KR, Broste SK, Frantz RP, Davis JM, Ringel A, Suchindran CM, Hibbeln JR. "Re-evaluation of the Traditional Diet-Heart Hypothesis: Analysis of Recovered Data from Minnesota Coronary Experiment (1968-73)." *BMJ* 2016; 353:i1246. bmj.com/content/353/bmj.i1246.full.pdf+html

Chapter 11: Anger Rising

should anyone question that again: Hallberg S, Campbell W, "Retrospective Analysis of Metabolic Control in Type 2 Diabetes with American Diabetes Association Recommendations compared with Carbohydrate Restriction." *Journal of Clinical Lipidology* Abstract 2015 May; 9(3): 420.

lipidjournal.com/article/S1933-2874(15)00113-0/fulltext

Chapter 14: Virta

before we had insulin and other medication: The Epilepsy Center. Johns Hopkins Medicine. "Timeline: Ketogenic Diet Therapy for Epilepsy | The Johns Hopkins Epilepsy Center. hopkinsmedicine.org/neurology_neurosurgery/centers_clinics/epilepsy/keto-diet-timeline.html

Chapter 15: Exhaustion, Recognition, Almost Perfection

all you could hope to do was manage it: Cefalu WT; Rubino F, Cummings DE. "Metabolic Surgery for Type 2 Diabetes: Changing the Landscape of Diabetes Care." *Diabetes Care* 2016; 39(6):857–860. doi.org/10.2337/dc16-0686

guidelines and diabetes reversal: Hallberg SJ, Dockter NE, Kushner JA, Athinarayanan SJ. "Improving the Scientific Rigour of Nutritional Recommendations for Adults with Type 2 Diabetes: A Comprehensive Review of the American Diabetes Association Guideline-Recommended Eating Patterns." *Diabetes, Obesity and Metabolism: A Journal of Pharmacology and Therapeutics* 2019 Aug; 21(8):1769-1779. doi.org/10.1111/dom.13736

Chapter 16: Before and After

published a few months earlier: McKenzie AL, Hallberg SJ, Creighton BC, Volk BM, Link TM, Abner MK, Glon RM, McCarter JP, Volek JS, Phinney SD. "A Novel Intervention Including Individualized Nutritional Recommendations Reduces Hemoglobin A1c Level, Medication Use, and Weight in Type 2 Diabetes." *JMIR Diabetes* 2017; 2(1):e5.
diabetes.jmir.org/2017/1/e5/

Chapter 17: Making the Best

one-year results for those with diabetes: Hallberg SJ, McKenzie AL, Williams PT, Bhanpuri NH, Peters AL, Campbell WW, Hazbun TL, Volk BM, McCarter JP, Phinney SD, Volek JS. "Effectiveness and Safety of a Novel Care Model for the Management of Type 2 Diabetes at 1 Year: An Open-Label, Non-Randomized, Controlled Study." *Diabetes Therapy* 2018 Feb 9:583-612.
link.springer.com/article/10.1007/s13300-018-0373-9

Chapter 18: Getting the Word Out

that of the White population: Centers for Disease Control and Prevention. "Native Americans with Diabetes: Better Diabetes Care Can Decrease Kidney Failure." *CDC Vital Signs* 1/10/17.
stacks.cdc.gov/view/cdc/43748

the biggest blockbuster in history: Tahir D. "Morning eHealth." *Politico*. 02/08/2018. politico.com/newsletters/morning-ehealth/2018/02/08/senate-reaches-wide-ranging-budget-deal-097047

cancers, respiratory, and especially diabetes: Swiss Re. "Solutions to address modifiable risks like type 2 diabetes." swissre.com/reinsurance/life-and-health/solutions/diabetes.html

was well over $300 billion: American Diabetes Association. *"Economic Costs of Diabetes in the U.S. in 2017." Diabetes Care 2018; 41(5):917–928.* diabetesjournals.org/care/article/41/5/917/36518/Economic-Costs-of-Diabetes-in-the-U-S-in-2017

Chapter 19: Bye Bye, Low Fat

we published our two-year results: Athinarayanan SJ, Adams RN, Hallberg SJ, McKenzie AL, Bhanpuri NH, Campbell WW, Volek JS, Phinney SD, McCarter JP. "Long-Term Effects of a Novel Continuous Remote Care Intervention Including Nutritional Ketosis for the Management of Type 2 Diabetes: A 2-Year Non-randomized Clinical Trial." *Frontiers in Endocrinology* 2019 Jun; 10:348. pubmed.ncbi.nlm.nih.gov/31231311/

participants who were prediabetic: McKenzie AL, Athinarayanan SJ, McCue JJ, Adams RN, Keyes M,

McCarter JP, Volek JS, Phinney SD, Hallberg SJ. "Type 2 Diabetes Prevention Focused on Normalization of Glycemia: A Two-Year Pilot Study." *Nutrients* 2021 Mar; 13(3):749.
ncbi.nlm.nih.gov/pmc/articles/PMC7996820/

lower progression to type 2 diabetes: Cannon MJ, Masalovich S, Ng BP, Soler RE, Jabrah R, Ely EK, Smith BD. "Retention Among Participants in the National Diabetes Prevention Program Lifestyle Change Program, 2012–2017." *Diabetes Care* 2020; 43:2042–2049.
diabetesjournals.org/care/article/43/9/2042/35791/

Ely EK, Gruss SM, Luman ET, Gregg EW, Ali MK, Nhim K, Rolka DB, Albright AL. "A National Effort to Prevent Type 2 Diabetes: Participant-Level Evaluation of CDC's National Diabetes Prevention Program." *Diabetes Care* 2017; 40(10):1331-1341.
diabetesjournals.org/care/article/40/10/1331/29533/A-National-Effort-to-Prevent-Type-2-Diabetes

Perreault L, Pan Q, Mather KJ, Watson KE, Hamman RF, Kahn SE, MB ChB for the Diabetes Prevention Program Research Group. "Effect of Regression from Prediabetes to Normal Glucose Regulation on Long-Term Reduction in Diabetes Risk: Results from the Diabetes Prevention Program Outcomes Study." *The Lancet* 2012 Jun; 379(9833):2243-2251.
thelancet.com/journals/lancet/article/PIIS0140-6736(12)60525-X/fulltext

Knowler WC, Barrett-Connor E, Fowler SE, Hamman RF, Lachin JM, Walker EA, Nathan DM. "Reduction in the Incidence of Type 2 Diabetes with Lifestyle Intervention or Metformin." N. Engl. *J. Med.* 2002; 346:393–403.
nejm.org/doi/full/10.1056/nejmoa012512

the unfounded vilification of saturated fat: Nutrition Coalition. "'Miracle' Conference in Zurich." June 23, 2018. nutritioncoalition.us/news/food-for-thought-conference/

a real turning point: Davies MJ, D'Alessi DA, Fradkin J, Kernan WN, Mathieu C, Mingrone G, Rossing P, Tsapas A, Wexler DJ, Buse JB. "Management of Hyperglycemia in Type 2 Diabetes, 2018. A Consensus Report by the American Diabetes Association (ADA) and the European Association for the Study of Diabetes (EASD). *Diabetes Care* 2018; 41(12):2669–2701.
diabetesjournals.org/care/article/41/12/2669/36544/Management-of-Hyperglycemia-in-Type-2-Diabetes

including low-carb choices: Evert AB, Dennison M, Gardner CD, Garvey WT, Lau KHK, MacLod J, Mitri J, Pereira RF, Rawlings K, Robinson S, Saslow L, Uelmen S, Urbanski PB, Yancy Jr WS. "Nutrition Therapy for Adults With Diabetes or Prediabetes: A Consensus Report." *Diabetes Care* 2019; 42(5):731–754. doi.org/10.2337/dci19-0014

American Diabetes Association. "Lifestyle Management: Standards of Medical Care in Diabetes—

2019." *Diabetes Care* 2019; 42 (Supplement_1):S46–S60. doi.org/10.2337/dc19-S005

citing three of our papers: Merril JD, Soliman D, Kumar N, Lim S, Shariff AI, Yancy, Jr. WS. "Low-Carbohydrate and Very-Low-Carbohydrate Diets in Patients With Diabetes." *Diabetes Spectrum* 2020; 33(2):133–142. doi.org/10.2337/ds19-0070

Made in the USA
Coppell, TX
08 May 2024

32017579R00174